Acupuncture
T A I L S

A Vet's Story
of Treating Animals
& Their Owners

Best wishes, Jane Hunter

By
Jane EB Hunter
BVMS PhD MRCVS DipMedAc UHCert

Acupuncture Tails: A Vet's Story of Treating Animals and their Owners
© Jane EB Hunter 2021 All rights reserved.
Published by JEB Hunter (an imprint of Swan & Horn Publishers) 2021
Website: www.janeebhunter.vet

Printed version ISBN 978-1-909675-27-8
Kindle version ISBN 978-1-909675-28-5
Createspace version ISBN 978-1-909675-29-2
Audio version ISBN 978-1-909675-30-8

The book contains the real names of the pets and humans treated by the Author, with their kind permission. Some names have been changed where it has not been possible to obtain their permission, or as requested by their owners. The Author does not represent any society and all observations, interpretations and comments are her own (unless otherwise stated). The Author recommends obtaining medical or veterinary advice before seeking acupuncture.

Editorial, design & production by Maria Carter and Sophie Hampshire (www.swanandhorn.com)
Production assistant Hannah Phillips
Cover illustrator Shona M'gadzah
Printed by The Evolve Group (www.theevolvegroup.co.uk)

Praise for *Tails*

From the animal tales ...

"When my Spaniel Oz was nearly put to sleep due to his unmanageable back pain – having exhausted all the painkiller options – we tried it. He was restored and we are forever grateful"

"We were amazed when our Yorkshire Terrier Kizi – who had a liver condition – improved to the extent that she didn't need frequent hospitalisation!"

"Sometimes it feels as though the benefits of Petra's acupuncture session extend beyond the dog herself – with such a tactile treatment and all of us being hands on, there is definitely the sense of a communal experience."

And the human tales ...

"When I saw how mobile and full of energy my Labrador Oscar was after starting acupuncture for his osteoarthritis, I wanted to try it for myself – it has really helped me cope with my polymyalgia and reduced the need for so much medication (for us both)."

"I was worried I would become hooked on opiates again; now I only need to take occasional medication – a weight has been lifted off me and I'm getting great nights' sleep."

"After 18 months with practically no sense of smell or taste, I felt miserable – until there was an almost immediate return with acupuncture. After a few sessions I got them back 95% and I'm so happy! My ENT consultant was amazed!"

"The relief from the headaches I got from acupuncture helped me think more clearly – therefore I could reassess my job and lifestyle and make changes."

To something for all ...

"Definitely inspiring and great to read about real cases and the effect of acupuncture on real lives, rather than the constant cold emotionless numbers from trials and statistics."
Duncan Lawler—Consultant physiotherapist and acupuncturist, Chair of British Medical Acupuncture Society (BMAS) Professional Services & author of Western Medical Acupuncture Protocols for Chronic Pain

This book is dedicated to
my four-legged and two-legged patients
(and three-legged Tweak!) past and present –
it has been a privilege to know them.

A percentage of the proceeds from the sale of this book
will be donated to the charity Mission Rabies.

Find out more here

www.missionrabies.com

"The key is to stay open to all possibilities and I tell my kids that. I tell them 'Beware of people who know the answer. Seek the company of people who are trying to understand the question. Stay open and you will find that you're drawn to things naturally.' A lot of people miss mountains of things that could make their lives lovely. If they don't go out and try something, they'll miss out."

Billy Connolly, comedian and author
of *Journey to the Edge of the World*

Contents

Acknowledgements

Iam indebted to all the pet owners and human patients for letting me share their stories and their support and enthusiasm. To use owner Ellen's words about her Border Collie Petra's acupuncture, "it has certainly been a communal experience". As for the four-legged stars, I think most wouldn't mind the attention.

A big thank you goes to all the referring vets in my local area and the vets, doctors and staff at Albavet, St Clair and Millhill surgeries, where my clinics were held, for their support and friendship along the way. Particular thanks to Rachel Rogers of Inglis Vets, Jarlath Busby and Ian Paterson at St Clair Vet Group (Ian also willingly offered his photographs), and Angus Mcpherson of Lomond Hills Vet Clinic; also Ann Hutchison at Dalblair Vets, who was encouraging from the start and always willing to share her vast knowledge and expertise on the role of acupuncture in veterinary practice, and also of treating people. Special thanks go to the British Medical Acupuncture Society (BMAS) for their training and help over the years, especially medical director Mike Cummings and my BMAS Diploma mentor, Val Dudgeon; and to my friend and colleague, and fellow BMAS member, GP Liz Phillips, senior partner at Millhill Surgery, without whom so much of this would have been impossible. I'm forever indebted for your advice, caring and sharing – and the cycling!

To all the people who read all (or bits and pieces) of the manuscript, thank you, too, for your time and input. I was lucky to find Maria Carter of Swan & Horn – your enthusiasm, commitment and attention to detail have been amazing in seeing *Tails* through to publication!

I'd also like to thank Beth Cruickshank and my school friend Alison Cooper, for always being supportive and providing a constant stream of family, friends and occupational therapists for treatment!

And last but not least, I am forever grateful to my very patient husband, Kenneth, for his love and unwavering support.

There are many tales missing from this book – apologies to those that 'got away', but thank you all for being there.

1

Figures in this book

Fig. 1 The Gall Bladder (GB) channel showing four commonly used points. Courtesy of Dr Mike Cummings.

Fig. 2 The skeleton of a human.

Fig. 3 The skeleton of a dog.

Fig. 4 A map of Bryan's head pain.

Fig. 5 A map of Bryan's neck and shoulder pain.

Fig. 6 A map of Lynsey's head pain.

Fig. 7 A map of Scott's pain located by massage.

Fig. 8 A map of George's leg pain associated with plantar fasciitis.

Fig. 9 The World Small Animal Veterinary Association's (WSAVA) body condition score chart for dogs.

Photo credits

Ian Paterson for all photographs in Chapter 1 and of Suilven in Chapter 2.

Kristeen Barker for the photograph of Ben in Chapter 3.

Lisa Grice for the photograph of Guinness in Chapter 10.

Kevin Smith for the photograph of Flora in Chapter 14.

Jackie and Alan Ogilvie for the photographs of Paolo in Chapter 15.

Shona Hedley for the photograph of Pickles in the Epilogue.

Shona M'Gadzah for the cover illustration.

Joyce Henderson for the photograph of the Author.

Foreword

Dr Liz Phillips
MB BS BScHons DRCOG

Jane has been a friend and colleague since 2004, when she approached my GP practice in search of a room for treating acupuncture patients. At that point, she had received massage and acupuncture training, on top of her vet and PhD degrees, and through working in academia and vet practice she was experienced in delivering a caring service. As a GP and a member of the British Medical Acupuncture Society (BMAS) myself, this arrangement was an excellent fit as I felt there was a place for more acupuncture in healthcare for humans. In 2006, Jane was awarded the BMAS Diploma in Western Medical Acupuncture – the only vet to complete it, as far as I know.

Although I have been around for many of the events in this book, and during its writing, the final book has still been a joy to read. Jane's high level of empathy and humanity shines through the stories she tells, and the pets pop out of the pages as 'friends'. Readers will become truly invested in their lives and trials. Jane saw many human patients during her time at my surgery, all of whom valued the methods she employed to support their healthcare journey and improve their lives.

Acupuncture Tails shows how humanity, combined with science, can have beneficial outcomes for all patients – two-legged, four-legged and even three-legged. This book will captivate all those with an interest in healthcare and pets; after all, there are similar treatment options for them and us mere humans.

I can honestly say that being involved with Jane's book has brought back the joy of acupuncture as a tool in my medical arsenal, and as life begins to return to normal during the long global coronavirus pandemic, I hope to soon reintroduce it for my patients. Thank you, Jane, for this beautiful reminder of how art and science come together in our daily practice.

Preface

The true tales in this book are by way of a celebration of the help acupuncture has given my human, canine and feline patients over the past twenty-one years. These are my own words and interpretations and do not represent any society or other organisation. Permission to share these stories was very willingly given by the owners, patients and relatives. Names have been changed if someone has not been traceable and to respect privacy where requested.

While the evidence for the effectiveness of acupuncture treatment carried out in published trials is eagerly sought, and the results continue to be debated by the medical profession, I believe it is also still important to record the case histories and observations of treating individual cases in the clinic.

For readers who haven't experienced acupuncture, I would urge you to find out about it for yourself or your pet when in need – and then you can make up your own mind. I also recommend that you obtain medical or veterinary advice before seeking acupuncture.

Prologue

Staying in New Zealand for just over the mandatory three years, I became a citizen. I was keeping my options open, believing that leaving academia and going back home was right for me. After all, I was now a *Scottish* Kiwi and could always return to New Zealand if I made the wrong decision. But, much as I loved the Land of the Long White Cloud, I was *too* Scottish, *too* far away from home, family and old friends. I knew I'd miss my Kiwi ones, especially Sheryll and Rosie and their families, but I had met some Brits who had not settled completely in New Zealand, and they had been there for so long that the UK wasn't home for them either. And what if anyone in my family became unwell? I'd seen the dilemmas faced by some of my colleagues and I didn't want that to happen to me. So, in 1999 I headed back to Fife, taking a slow route west.

My first stop was Tasmania and the Australian Veterinary Conference, where I planned to meet up with my friend Barb. We had both been lecturers at Massey University, the only vet school in New Zealand. She was a pig vet and had left to take up a job in Australia. I had been a lecturer in veterinary bacteriology and had no idea what my next job would be. All I knew was I wanted to work with my hands on live animals again.

After graduating from Glasgow University Veterinary School in 1983, I spent five years in mainly small animal practices, including working and travelling in Australia. I never wanted the commitment of having my own practice, and the combination of curiosity and opportunity led to me gaining my PhD in 1992 in antibiotic resistance from Liverpool University.

Based at both the vet school and Royal Liverpool Hospital, I had the broad remit of looking at the possible transfer of antibiotic resistance between animals and humans. I have always been fascinated with the animal–human relationship and our place together in the world, so while it was a far cry from hands-on practice, it gave me a different perspective. Next came a few months of campaigning against the transport of live animals in Europe, followed by three years working as a veterinary investigation officer, diagnosing diseases of mainly farm animals, including post-mortem work. Somehow this led to my post as a senior lecturer in Veterinary Bacteriology in New Zealand.

Attending conferences had become a bit of a habit over those years, but the difference was that I had paid the conference fee for this latest one, in Tasmania, myself. The timing and location fitted in with meeting up with Barb, and we arrived in Hobart after a few days exploring Tasmania's beautiful east coast. Barb was giving a lecture and had all the 'pig talks' circled on the event list that she intended going to, but what was I doing there? I looked again at the list of topics and realised I'd had my fill of bacteria and dead things – I'd just been to a lecture about an unusual fungal infection in dogs following some orthopaedic operations. The fungus was described in intricate detail, but I was disappointed that the key question – why it had been able to cause infection in the first place? – was left unanswered.

I was struck by a block of lectures on Chinese medicine. This topic seemed incongruous, and I was instantly both curious and sceptical. This was a national veterinary conference so why was it being included? I knew it wouldn't have been back in the UK, due to a lack of 'evidence' in the area. However, the guest speaker delivering the session, one Dr Allen Schoen, had been invited from America by the Australian Association of Veterinary Acupuncturists. His lectures were spread over several days. My interest was piqued.

As the large auditorium filled up with vets, I became more and more uncomfortable in my seat. It wasn't just the heat. I knew nothing about acupuncture or Chinese herbal medicine and I didn't understand any of it. When it came to herbal medicine, the fact that some plants were toxic had put me off straight away. But acupuncture was different. It was a physical treatment.

The idea of inserting needles into animals, that they would show no discomfort, and that it was a form of veterinary treatment that could help with pain and a host of conditions, made me feel alienated. I had no idea what the speaker meant by 'meridians'. What and where were all the points he mentioned? Like LI4 which stood for Large Intestine 4 – this was weird! Despite my fifteen years in the veterinary profession – and the fact that only vets were allowed to treat animals with acupuncture – I knew little about its use in veterinary or human medicine.

In New Zealand I had a friend who had found instant relief with acupuncture treatment of a football injury. He had enjoyed elaborating on the length of the needle and where it had been placed. And I vaguely remembered a visiting lecturer at Glasgow Vet School who talked about acupuncture. That was in my final year but, because the subject wasn't examinable, I had not attended. I felt guilty now. I was being told this was a procedure that did no harm, and was in some cases life-changing – and life-saving. Dr Schoen was an expert in his field who had written textbooks on Chinese medicine and one that included his personal account of acupuncture. He had treated animals belonging to the rich and famous in the USA, where no expense was spared on diagnosis and conventional treatment, but sometimes it was acupuncture that made all the difference.

I was fascinated, but wondered why the animals tolerated it? Should I consider it for animals under my care if I went back into practice? Would it work for me? With my academic background, I wondered what scientific evidence there was for acupuncture. My naysayer voice was protesting loudly. According to the Cambridge English dictionary, a naysayer is 'someone who says something is not possible, is not good, or will fail'. That was me alright.

Going out that evening in Hobart with Dr Schoen and some other delegates, I was invited to visit a practice in Perth to see acupuncture in action. I jumped at the chance. Coincidentally, Barb's place in Perth was the last stop on my Australian itinerary. It all fell into place but I had no idea I was cementing a future career change.

Among the cases I saw in Perth, a large version of a German Shepherd called Max willingly walked on to a lowered tabletop, stood still while it was elevated, and then allowed the vet to insert needles along his spine and hips. As the owner fondled Max's ears, they chatted to the vet about Max's progress and how well he was coping since starting a course of acupuncture for hip dysplasia. A window in my mind was opening up to an entirely new approach for the management of mobility and pain.

In addition, Barb and I attended a meeting of the Australian Integrative Medicine Association. I had never heard of the description of integrative medicine. To explain, it's best to use their words from their website:

"Integrative medicine is a philosophy of healthcare with a focus on individual patient care. It combines the best of conventional western medicine with evidence-based complementary medicine and therapies. [It] reaffirms the importance of the relationship between practitioner and patient, focuses on the whole person, is informed by evidence, and makes use of all appropriate therapeutic approaches, healthcare professionals and disciplines to achieve optimal health and healing. It takes into account the physical, psychological,

social and spiritual wellbeing of the person with the aim of using the most appropriate, safe and evidence-based treatments available."

What I had learned about massage and what I thought acupuncture was all about seemed to come under this umbrella of integrative medicine and resonated strongly with me – for both humans and animals.

It all set me on a mission. In 1999 I was planning to return to clinical work in small animal practice in Scotland and somehow learn about acupuncture. I had no idea how it would go down, but it is no doubt due to my chance experiences in Australia that I am writing my own acupuncture tales twenty-one years later.

— 1 —

Vetting 'down under'

In 1987, after three years' experience of small animal practice as a veterinary surgeon in the UK, I answered an advert for a six-month job in a mixed practice in Berri, South Australia.

I had spent a few weeks in Australia before, back in 1985, to visit a boyfriend, and I knew I would be back. It was such a fascinating country. The first time flying over the vastness of the inner continent and Ayers Rock etched the vivid red colour of the land into my memory, but none more so than the spectacular hues of the crimson rosellas around the bird feeders in the garden. This time, I had longer to spend there, with an Australian visa for a whole year, and with travel planned either side of work.

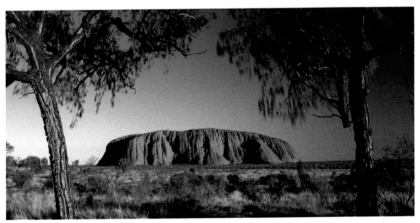

The awesome Uluru – the Aboriginal name for Ayers Rock.

I learned a lot in the Berri practice about many of the venomous creatures that the holiday brochures fail to mention. We had to be careful when walking in the countryside because of snakes. The advice was to avoid bare legs and to stamp your feet to scare them away. Several dogs were admitted to the practice after being bitten by snakes. The venoms of the black or king-brown snakes contained a powerful neurotoxin that caused respiratory paralysis. It was standard practice to anaesthetise the affected dog as soon as possible and administer antivenom intravenously. Sometimes it was successful, other times not. Cats were different. They simply became paralysed and floppy, were given antivenom and hospitalized on a drip – and would recover within a few days.

While the practice was mixed – with horses, cows and the occasional wildlife case like an orphaned kangaroo with diarrhoea – my role was mainly to deal with small animals. I was uneasy around horses, and after the night I drove a hundred and twenty miles to calve a cow in a storm – with the rotten calf coming away in pieces as the mother had been 'out bush' for some days, everything covered in sand and the farmer cracking James Herriot jokes – I doubted my future lay in mixed practice!

With temperatures approaching fifty degrees Celsius, the Riverland area around Berri and by the Murray River was so desert-like that I longed to be among rolling green hills instead. So, when my job ended, my travels began. First on the list was a guided river-rafting, cycling and hill-walking holiday, starting in Launceston, Tasmania.

Seeing the yellow-tailed black cockatoos (straight out of the pages of my bird book) cawing overhead as we approached Dove Lake in Cradle Mountain National Park blew me away! While some of the scenery could have been Scotland, the wallabies on the beach and these cockatoos reminded me I was half-way round the world. I had no more on-call work, no long-distance drives, and no need to deal with 'vet stuff' … but of course there is never an escape.

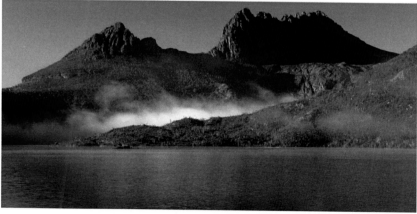

Dove Lake and Cradle Mountain – home to yellow-tailed black cockatoos.

Blue's sore eye

Our party had just arrived at a farm stay when I spied a big shaggy farm dog, a bit like an Old English Sheepdog, and while the other dogs bounded around, he sat quietly with one eye closed. I knew he would have little chance of being taken to a vet, so I asked the farmer if I could try to examine him.

Blue sat still as I approached slowly. I had no idea of his temperament and with my training I'm always prepared for a surprise, no matter how cute and cuddly the animal's appearance. He allowed me to stroke his head and I could see how matted his grey curly hair was around his eye, and how bloodshot the tiny visible part of the cornea was behind the swollen and seeping eyelids. My heart sank. He had been like this for some time.

I felt encouraged as Blue continued to sit patiently and allowed me to lift his upper eyelid, just far enough to see a huge piece of grass wedged there. With no sedative or equipment handy, or even local anaesthetic eye drops, what could I do? I needed help, so I asked Shona, one of the holiday guides. She came back with a pair of tweezers and volunteered to hold him. I felt totally responsible for her safety, but Blue continued to sit with Shona holding his head as I took a closer look. Could I remove the grass entirely? I might make it worse if he struggled or jumped and the tweezers poked his eye. Taking a deep breath, as Shona held him firmly, I grasped the stem of the grass in the middle of his eye, willing him to keep still. As a one-inch strand came out complete, I felt the warm inner glow of satisfaction. Then Blue skipped off with what must have been instant relief, as Shona and I hugged each other.

On my return to the UK in 1988, I was back in practice for a few months, but I felt restless with its constraints. The traditional idea of being a vet is working in practice, not necessarily James Herriot-style nowadays, but treating animals nonetheless. However, there are many other opportunities for vets – government jobs with the Home Office, disease investigation, meat and food hygiene, various avenues in veterinary and medical research, academic roles in veterinary schools, and specialisms within clinical practice and wildlife. While I was thinking about some kind of career change, a vet friend, who had not long started studying for a PhD, suggested I apply for a similar opening at Liverpool University. So came the leap into academia –

and the topic of antibiotic resistance. A steep learning curve, and just the first of many to follow. I was re-introduced to the world of bacteria, specifically the ones that live in the guts of pigs and humans. There were a few eureka moments. Resistance to some aminoglycoside antibiotics, used in both animals and humans, was found on plasmids – genetic material that can be transferred from one bacterium to another. And I was able to show that it was present on some pigs in some pig farms, and on calves too, as well as the pig workers. And on the beef in one butcher's shop.

After my PhD I became a veterinary investigation (VI) officer back in Scotland. Then, after three years of farm-animal post-mortem and diagnostic work, I found myself back in the Southern Hemisphere.

The Land of the Long White Cloud, Aotearoa 1994

Feeling out of place in the VI service and needing a different perspective on life, my cousin and I planned a big trip to New Zealand. I had free rein to design a four-week tour exploring the North and South Islands, to see some of the unique wildlife. Cousin Marjorie was happy to go anywhere. Tiritiri Matangi Island, off the coast of Auckland, was a great start, a haven created for the native birds, safe from introduced predators like rats, possums and cats.

Uncannily, just before we were due to leave for New Zealand, a job was advertised in the *Veterinary Record*, the journal of the British Veterinary Association. It was for a lecturing post at Massey University in Palmerston North, New Zealand. Did I have the qualifications? What if I did? Would I go? It was an effort to create an up-to-date CV, but I went ahead and applied. The result was an informal interview, specially scheduled between Christmas and the New Year, towards the end of my holiday.

Like Australia, New Zealand is a wonderful country to explore and many of the native species are unique. The marine life is special, boasting the world's smallest dolphin, Hector's dolphin, which can only be seen in certain areas. And if you are lucky, and weather permitting, you may see sperm whales at Kaikoura. The Otago Peninsula near Dunedin is the only mainland nesting site for royal albatrosses. Fur seals and yellow-eyed penguins (*overpage*) can be found nearby.

The black stilts at Twizel are a species fighting against habitat change, but the flightless takahe, that were thought to be extinct in the 1950s,

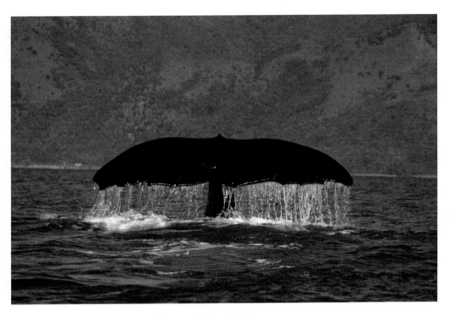

Sperm whale at Kaikoura.

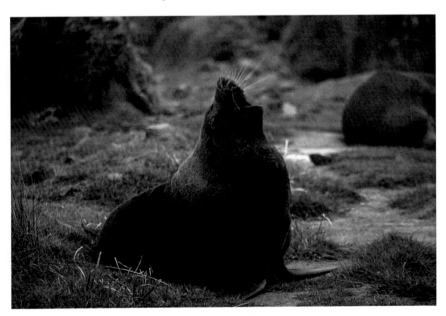

Fur seal at the Otago Peninsula.

have made a comeback under the careful management of the Department of Conservation. It was disappointing that the only kiwis we saw were in captivity, and it was a bit disturbing to see an advert for the 'Great Alexandra Bunny Shoot', a competition to see how many rabbits can be shot by a team of hunters in twenty-four hours.

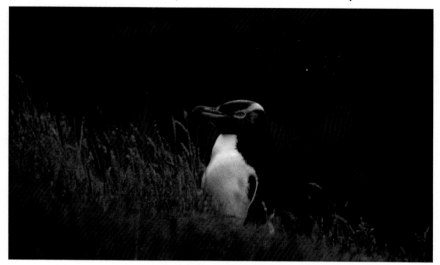

A Hoi Hoi, the Maori name for the yellow-eyed penguin.

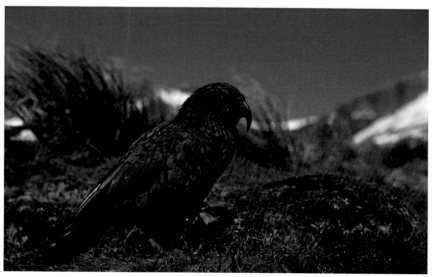

A kea, the 'mountain parrot' found on the South Island.

Walking the Milford track over four days was stunning. I had a moment of clarity at the Mackinnon Pass, when I knew I would be leaving my diagnostic pathology job back in the UK, whether I was coming to New Zealand or not. I was a square peg in a round hole, even if I was glad to be living in Scotland again after my shorter spells of working in Kent and Cheshire and my PhD days in Liverpool.

A paragraph from the book by Malachy Tallack called *Sixty Degrees North*, about his travels through countries in that latitude, resonated with me. He talked of his curiosity to explore and his restlessness, describing the latter as:

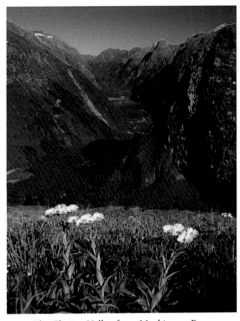

The Clinton Valley from Mackinnon Pass.

'that joy and curse that I have known for most of my life, brings unease when I ought to be content: it brings contentment when I ought to be uneasy. It sends me out into the world, almost against my will'.

I was amazed when, on my return to Scotland, I was offered the post in New Zealand. Getting a visa was not easy though. I had to write to all of my bosses over the previous eleven years to prove I was eligible, by scoring enough points. I also had to get medicals done and numerous documents validated.

Academia New-Zealand style 1995–1999

I arrived back in New Zealand in August 1995 to join the Department of Veterinary Pathology and Public Health at Massey University, amidst the pall of the All Blacks losing the Rugby World Cup Final to South Africa. I quickly learned not to mention it.

It was supposedly winter, but at sixteen degrees Celsius (sixty-one Fahrenheit) the days would pass as summertime in Scotland. Shorts and t-shirt weather, but strangely the outdoor swimming pool was closed for the season. The university arranged accommodation in a motel for my first three weeks. At the end of my stay, the owner Val who ran it told me I had surprised her. She had expected this Dr Hunter to be male, aged and likely sporting a grey beard – not female, in her thirties, carrying a rucksack.

Starting to lecture in veterinary bacteriology without any training in how to do it was a steep learning curve for me. After the first lecture I gave, I stood on a chair to remove my slides. The chair shook, and I turned to see who was making it move. No one. It was my first earthquake. Something I never got used to in all the time I was there. The ground shook on a regular basis. Kiwis simply accept that they live on a fault line. It was why there was a notice up at the entrance to our building – what to do in the event of an earthquake, a volcanic eruption, or tsunami … I didn't know then that a tsunami was a massive tidal wave usually caused by seismic activity.

One of my earliest tasks in the department was not academic. When I told my father over the phone, he wondered why a lecturer was organising the installation of more toilets. I was only the second female lecturer in the department, and the first senior one. Changes were afoot, because the number of female students had been increasing, but not the number of toilets. The female students were often late for lectures because they had to queue for so long for the sparse facilities. No one was sorting it out, so I felt I had to. I should have expected that I would often get side-tracked, and in ways I could never imagine.

Settling in was made easier due to the friendly staff who were used to others coming and going, and also because there was a Celtic–Polish contingent already there. My bacteriology colleague was Stan, also a Glasgow graduate. He was well established and very entertaining, often using photographs of his time in Yemen to illustrate his lectures. Joanne and Colin, head of our section, were virologists, so the four of us lectured on infectious diseases. That seems a luxury now with the cutbacks on staffing levels within universities, but we were kept busy with our research in addition to teaching and setting exams – computers were only slowly beginning to appear!

At least in practice, the day would come to an end, but the ways we could contribute to university life were never-ending. To balance my academic life early on I went on a bushcraft weekend where I met Rosie, our Kiwi leader. She and her family became great friends of mine and integrated me into true Kiwi life. When I first went to Rosie's house, which she was sharing at the time, I don't know who was more surprised – I was introduced to her housemates only to find they were three of my Massey vet students!

I had many fascinating things to learn about – both good and bad. Possums introduced for the New Zealand fur trade now ran rampant through the country, and multiplied into the millions, drastically reducing the native bird population. They also carry TB, another zoonotic bacterium that can spread from animals to humans. Some animal disease-causing bacterial strains differ from those in the UK. Leptospirosis, for example, is an important disease affecting farmed deer, and is also zoonotic, largely due to a pig strain – not a cow strain as in the UK. The *Campylobacter* bacterium is a major source of food poisoning compared to the UK, due to the Kiwis' love of barbecues – and their inadvertent eating of undercooked chicken.

In my lectures I described the type of bacterium and its specific properties, the conditions it needed to multiply, how it spread, the types of disease it caused and gave an understanding of the steps that could be taken to prevent the disease. The zoonotic diseases were the most interesting to me, and I was able to demonstrate their global nature and the importance of hygiene. I showed the students a film about an outbreak of *Escherichia coli* O157 in a butcher's shop near Wishaw in Scotland. There were practical classes, too, on how to culture and identify bacteria, such as harmless versions of *E. coli,* using a microscope and specific chemical reactions. When I suggested the students draw the letter A, for example, using their finger on a culture plate to demonstrate how many bacteria lived on their hands, many drew the outline of an E – my accent was a constant source of amusement! On the university's annual Student's Day, it was unexpected (and fun) to be the 'kidnapped' academic; some final-year students turned up at my house early in the morning and I was more than surprised to be taken abseiling and made to wear an outfit provided by them for their '60s disco.

In the office next door to mine there were two lecturers in veterinary public health. They dealt with commercial slaughter, meat inspection, hygiene and safety. Their research topic caught my interest straight away – they were trying to highlight the inhumane methods used for slaughtering whales, in a bid to stop it happening.

Because I had worked in the VI service in Scotland, I knew that marine mammals that were found dead were reported and, if possible, taken into a VI centre so that records could be kept about the species and causes of death. Being in southeast Scotland at the time, I had only dealt with a few cases; most of the work was carried out at the Inverness centre, largely on the famous local populations of bottlenose dolphins and harbour porpoises. I assumed there must be a 'strandings' protocol in New Zealand, too, because of its wealth of marine life and huge coastline, but there was no system in place. The Department of Conservation is a government body that acts as their wildlife guardian, who occasionally sent a marine carcass to the university – but it was pot luck whether it went to the anatomists, who studied the anatomical differences between species, or the pathologists, who examined cause of death.

Our application for funding was successful for a strandings project, and this led to the arrival of Padraig, a post-doctoral marine mammal vet, who had completed a PhD on a viral disease in seals. Since then, a lot has changed. Massey University has established a dedicated Wildlife Centre; and Padraig is now the chief research pathologist at the Marine Mammal Center in California.

I had to adapt to the academic way of life and working with students. Exam time was an eye-opener for me, picking through some awful English to spot correct answers. Some of the mature students were around my age, but I realised how much older I was than them, in the way we dressed, for example, and how much had changed since I had graduated in 1983. I felt decidedly uncomfortable sitting with the Professor during the oral examinations; one student arrived in shorts, a holey vest, holey socks and a knitted tammy (there were probably holes in that, too).

When I was a student in Glasgow, some of the boys were sent away from the examination room to smarten up – a collar and tie were essential. At Massey, the senior staff had long debates about how to tell a female fourth-year student that wearing elbow-length black gloves was not appropriate in the clinic – it was impossible for her to do the job properly! It should have been straightforward, a matter of hygiene, and hands needed to be washed between patients. In contrast, my very good friend Sheryll, who became personal assistant to the Dean, and one of her colleagues gave a final-year student a very hard time.

They had been totally honest with him, saying they wouldn't want to take a pet to him because his face was covered in piercings; it was unprofessional, they said, and told him he should be more concerned about the animals than his appearance – laying it on far more strongly than any faculty staff member would have done.

In some ways, my time in New Zealand felt like stepping back in time – there were no ready-cooked meals in the supermarket, for instance, but in other ways it felt like stepping into the future. They had bank-card chips and PINs then, in 1995, around ten years before the UK, and they had been identifying sheep using bar codes on tags for even longer. There was an excellent after-hours medical drop-in service open from six to ten on weekday evenings, something that would take a lot of pressure off after-hours services and GP appointments in the NHS. My mother had received prompt attention from the drop-in service for an acute bout of cystitis when she was staying with me. Ironically, the doctor later guessed she was an overseas visitor from the results of her urine culture. The bacteria in it were multi-resistant, with a pattern of resistance to some commonly used antibiotics – unlike what you'd normally find in the urine of Kiwis with cystitis!

I seemed to go through a pattern of change around every three years in my career. When I look back, I can see each one as a stepping-stone. After my three years in New Zealand, I felt I had to leave, or else I might never leave! As I said, I felt too Scottish, too far from home, and – most importantly – I didn't want to stay in academia. The seventh floor of Massey felt like an 'ivory tower'. Fascinating as infectious diseases and diseased tissues are, I couldn't face writing another research-grant application, especially as so many more researchers were trying to get money from an ever-decreasing pot. Meanwhile, my hands had become 'twitchy'. Everything I was working with was dead.

Massage and touch

So much of being a vet is about touching, and I began to realise how much I missed the touch and response of a live animal. Because an animal obviously can't use words to tell us how they feel, vets rely very much on examination and the art of palpation – using our hands, for example, to try to find the source of pain or discomfort, to spot differences in muscles and joints, to determine how significant a skin lump might be, or to feel the abdomen for tension or anything unusual inside. Curiosity got the better of me when I saw a course in complementary therapies at Manawatu Polytechnic, just across town, which I could do in the weekends and evenings. But this was for people – not animals! I was side-tracked yet again, but it led to a recognised qualification in 1997, in massage with tasters in aromatherapy and reflexology. I was so impressed by the 'feeling' massage gave – both in receiving and giving. I had no idea how much tension I'd been carrying in my own body, and had been totally unaware of many sore areas, skilfully found by a fellow trainee as we worked on each other.

The firm nodules in my lower back worried me initially. I thought only enlarged lymph nodes felt like that, which were usually due to infection or cancer. My worries were soon alleviated when I learned that they often cropped up where tight muscles lay beneath; mine, I suspected, were from lifting too many heavy animals over the years. Learning about massage made me realise that the 'alternative' therapies offered other ways of treating ourselves and others, on top of the huge array of medicines available. I was also taking yoga classes, run by one of the massage teachers, and I learned how good it feels to have a good stretch. I dabbled, too, with Buddhism and meditation. It seemed that Kiwis were far more open to these things.

Eventually I had to acknowledge I was being pulled in a different direction from academia and life in New Zealand. I needed to work with my hands again, on live animals, or possibly even people! And to reconnect with the treating and caring aspects of clinical work.

That is why in May 1999, on my way home to Scotland, I found myself sitting in an auditorium with dozens of Australian vets and my internal naysayer's voice, listening avidly to the talks on acupuncture.

— 2 —

Homecoming and training

I arrived in Scotland yet again a month later, back with my very accommodating parents in the former mining town of Cowdenbeath, ready to return to practice. I had been home twice in three years, tagging my visits onto a conference somewhere, but this visit felt different. It was so satisfying to arrive at Edinburgh airport and seeing the two Forth bridges. There are three now, of course, but crossing the Forth after a spell away always held great significance for me – crossing back into the Kingdom of Fife, back to friends and family. And this time, I had a brand-new second nephew.

The first day of July saw the inauguration of Donald Dewar in Edinburgh as Scotland's First Minister. And on the same day, a large van-load of my belongings arrived. Aside from unpacking, I made it into the city and climbed Scott's monument to share in the occasion. So much was changing and, as I looked from the top of the monument over the Forth to Fife, and the outline of the Bishop and Lomond Hills, I thought back to the early days before I became a vet.

Tweak—and what felt like my first 'on call'!

I was thirteen years old and just dropping off to sleep when Mum burst into my bedroom. Jolted awake, I tried to make sense of her words. "Jane! You'll need to come. The cat's leg's off!"

Tweak had been found at the bottom of the back stairs. I rushed to the first cold, damp, concrete step and descended into the darkness beneath the weak light. What was waiting at the bottom? Halfway down, the stairs turned a corner. The back door was on the chain, leaving just enough space to let the cats in and out. There was Tweak, curled up on the doormat. I slowly approached and was met by a low, unearthly growl as her glazed black eyes came into view. Through the gloom I could make out the blood matting her tortoiseshell fur, and her limp hind paw poking out in a strange position. She hissed as I gingerly got onto my knees beside her and spoke. Tentatively, I reached out and touched her head, between her ears. She didn't flinch, so I began to stroke her. After a few moments of tousling, I couldn't believe what I was hearing. She started to purr. I was stunned that I was able to comfort her. As she continued to purr, I saw the gap where her knee should have been, her white paw attached only by a sliver of bloody tissue.

Dad used a blanket to scoop her up gently, his hands cradling her from underneath. She didn't move but managed a small growl. I sat in the back of the car, Tweak in a basket beside me, talking and stroking her as we sped to the vet's through the dark. Mr Gray had answered our call and told us to take her straight to his house. On the way Mum, Dad and I tried to work out what had happened. A train was the most likely cause. The railway line ran along the embankment at the bottom of our garden, and Tweak smelt of diesel. She must have climbed the six-foot-high brick wall that surrounded the entire garden, broken glass set in concrete all along the top.

It was a huge relief to pull up at the vet's house as instructed and hand Tweak over to the person we hoped could mend her. My brother Ron and Gran were so anxious that they'd already called him to see if we had arrived. The vet would keep Tweak comfortable overnight and then see what he could do in the morning.

I was horrified to hear then that her leg was to be amputated, wondering how Tweak could manage on three legs. But Mr Gray assured us that she was well in herself and would manage just fine. Two days later she was back home, her stump in a bandage, hobbling a bit further every day as she adjusted to life on three legs.

However, there was another cause for panic. I was at home alone when the bandage fell off and was terrified the wound would burst open. I phoned Dad, who calmly asked if the leg was bleeding. Looking more closely, I could see the area of shaved hair, a neat row of stitches at the end of the stump – and no blood. All was intact. With his usual bank-manager common-sense (hardly 'common' of course, because it's often not!) Dad just said, "She'll be fine, then".

Tweak's accident had more of an impact on me than I realised at the time. I still remember it vividly. I learned a lot from it, and two years later, during work experience at school, I got my first taste of life as a vet, with Mr Gray in his clinic. Would I be able to learn everything he knew, take responsibility, and make a difference to the lives of animals, like he did? Could I become a vet?

Tweak lived to a grand old age, always holding her own with the other cats in the household. She was the only one who worked out how to chap on the letterbox of the front door. We never saw how she managed to do it, but she could get Mum out of bed in the middle of the night to let her in.

I appreciate what a neat job Mr Gray did on Tweak back then, despite the limited choice of anaesthetics and analgesics (virtually none, in fact). How much has changed in veterinary practice since the seventies. When he retired, his practice was taken over by husband-and-wife team, Ryan and Calder, and after a somewhat circuitous route I ended up as one of their employees, and an acupuncturist.

Locum work—1999

Myself and a group of hillwalking friends managed to fit in a week's trip to Ullapool and the mountains of Assynt, including my favourite, Suilven, before I started work in the summer of 1999.

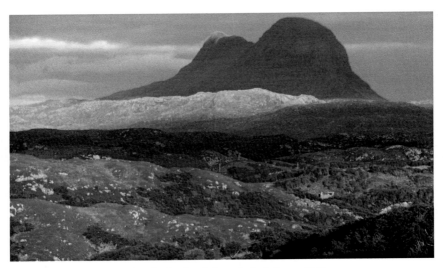

Back to Scotland and the majestic Suilven—1999.

I'd already been in touch with a classmate, Carol, who owned a busy small-animal practice in Barrhead in Renfrewshire and could give me some work over the summer. She had two young children, a schoolteacher husband, a horse and a dog and I had no idea how she juggled it all. I was in a completely different place from her, being single and starting all over again. After ten years out of clinical practice I can't say it was quite as nerve-racking as being a new graduate, but it was not far off.

Before I left New Zealand, I spent a few days operating in a friendly small-animal practice, doing some charity work and re-familiarising myself with the normal routines and procedures. I realised it's like riding a bike – you never forget. But you do lose confidence and speed, and I was all thumbs. I had to turn my ten thumbs back into dexterous fingers pretty quickly. I also volunteered at the SPCA in Fiji for a couple of weeks, working in very basic conditions, neutering dogs and re-honing my surgical skills.

One of the biggest changes in the UK after my ten-year absence was the increased use of broad-spectrum antibiotics. These drugs target a wide range of bacteria instead of specific ones, and are the same as those used in humans. Their use can be bad, though, because they contribute to antibiotic resistance and the rise of the 'superbugs' we hear so much about nowadays, making some diseases very hard to treat. For this reason, it's best to keep antibiotic use to a minimum, in both humans and animals. It's debatable how much their use in animals affects humans, but – as suggested by the concept of 'one health' – we are all inextricably linked. For these reasons, the medical and veterinary worlds now work together more closely.

This issue came up when I was studying for my PhD in Liverpool. I attended a talk on epidemiology one evening, where doctors and vets met up to present interesting cases of diseases and their diagnosis. The speaker was a veterinary professor of parasitology, and a sheep expert, whose friend suffered from a liver complaint that went undiagnosed, despite exhaustive testing. The professor said that if his friend had been a sheep, he would have diagnosed a liver-fluke infestation. These crop up in pastures contaminated by infected snails; the sheep eat them, the flukes grow inside them, then migrate to their livers, causing havoc.

The professor knew someone who worked in the hospital pathology department, who arranged for him to examine a biopsy of his friend's liver under the microscope. To the professor, the segments of flukes were clear to see but they had not been recognised by the medical staff, who had no experience in spotting sheep fluke. His friend was treated appropriately and made a good recovery. It turns out he had eaten some watercress picked from a contaminated pasture.

The importance of the 'one health' concept continues to grow. For example, the One Health Centre in Africa strives to improve the health of both humans and animals, as well as the local ecosystem, through networks that aim to control neglected zoonotic diseases, to understand emerging infectious diseases like the Covid-19 virus, to improve food safety, and to decrease antibiotic resistance. Alongside this, the World Health Organization (WHO) has set a target to eliminate dog-bite transmitted human deaths from rabies by 2030; and the charity Mission Rabies is doing its part to achieve this goal, by vaccinating dogs in a number of African and Asian countries. You can find out more about these organisations in the *Useful Links* section.

Acupuncture training in 1999

There was every chance that if I did not take up acupuncture quickly, my life and other work would take over. Acupuncture wasn't mainstream then, especially not for animals, and my idea could easily dissipate. I had to fit in the training somehow.

I kept scouring the *Veterinary Record* and one day there was a notice about an introductory course to be held during a weekend in November. It was run by Trixie Williams, a vet with a special interest in alternative therapies, and Dr David Dowson who, it later transpired, was also involved with the British Medical Acupuncture Society (BMAS). It was the only veterinary option I could find and when I made enquiries about it, I was surprised to be referred to BMAS. This charity was established in 1980 to train doctors and dentists, as well as vets. They now also offer training to nurses and allied health professionals, like osteopaths, chiropractors and, more recently, practitioners of traditional Chinese acupuncture. Usually their courses were held in the south of England but this foundation course was to be run in Glasgow, over two weekends. I signed up for it immediately, as well as a foundation course in homeopathy at Glasgow Homeopathic Hospital. I was going to learn about treating humans in both disciplines before doing a veterinary acupuncture course.

BMAS Foundation Course in Glasgow–September 1999

It was reassuring to see a face I recognised when I arrived at the venue in Glasgow. Mandy had been in the year above me at vet school and now owned a small-animal practice. She was feeling as out of her depth as I was. It may seem strange for vets to attend medical courses, but our pets are made of the same flesh and blood, with similar anatomy and diseases, so the results from human acupuncture can be adapted for use in them, as is the case for many medicines and procedures.

I didn't know there were different forms of acupuncture: from those based in traditional Chinese medicine (TCM) to western medical acupuncture (WMA). The latter aims to integrate acupuncture into conventional modern-day medicine, combining current knowledge of anatomy and physiology with scientific evidence. I was to discover there are many shades of grey in the area.

The course that day was led by Dr Mike Cummings, the Medical Director of BMAS. He had come into acupuncture through his military background, where he had first used it for musculoskeletal problems. There is plenty of information online now about the use of acupuncture, but here is a summary of what I first learned.

A wide variety of conditions can be treated with acupuncture, but it is especially effective for increasing mobility and reducing pain associated with sore joints and arthritis. Some palliative-care hospital units use it to alleviate symptoms like nausea and vomiting, as well as pain, and it's also useful for fertility issues and in childbirth.

The needles stimulate responses in the body that promote blood circulation, relax tense muscles and reduce pain and inflammation. There can be effects on the brain, too, with the release of hormones and feel-good factors that can bring about sleepiness and euphoria, sometimes described as a psychological boost.

The needles are usually made of stainless steel, and they are very fine, ranging from 0.16–0.4 millimetres in diameter, and 0.5–75 millimetres in length, depending on the area that's being treated. They have a plastic or metal hub, and the tips are smooth, like pencil tips – unlike the cutting edge of hypodermic needles used for injections. Because they have such a smooth shaft, infections from skin bacteria are rare. Previously the needles were considered to be reusable and they could, if improperly sterilised, transmit blood-borne viruses. Nowadays, there should be no cross-infections from needles between patients because they aren't reused, although they may be reinserted at different sites on a single patient, they are incinerated after use.

The fine straight needles are solid because nothing is injected through them, and when they are inserted into the skin or muscle their pencil-like tips simply *part* the tissue, rather than cutting them like a hypodermic needle. A local 'needle flare' reaction may occur where the skin surrounding the needle becomes red due to changes in circulation, or there may be 'needle grasp' if a muscle tightens around the needle. If a muscle contracts first then releases its tension quickly, the shaft can be bent, as shown here.

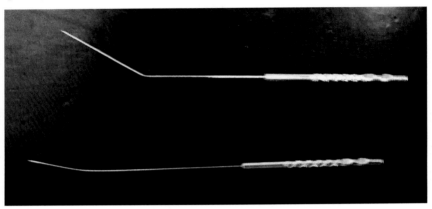

Muscle contraction can cause the needle shaft to bend.

The 'dose' of acupuncture relates to the number of needles used, the depth of insertion, how long the needles are in place for, and whether they are manipulated or just left there. The patient's response depends on how sensitive they are. Some people are 'strong' reactors and others 'weak'. Usually three or four sessions are recommended to begin with, but some conditions do better with five to twelve. Then again, sometimes one can be enough!

Acupuncture diagrams usually show six paired meridians, or channels – one at the front of the body and one at the back. There are many more than this, and they are annotated with numbered points, pretty much like a road atlas. Fig. 1 (*overpage*) shows the Gall Bladder (GB) channel, and several points along it. GB21 is often used to treat neck and shoulder pain and headaches, and GB30 is for pain that affects the hips and buttocks. Note that Gall Bladder is the name of the channel and has nothing to do with the actual gallbladder.

When it came to finding these points on the body, I was impressed to see how a point locator device was used. They are in zones of the skin where there is an increase in electrical conductivity due to low impedance of the skin. The point locator beeps when it finds a suitable site.

In the 1970s and 1980s, Western doctors like Felix Mann and Anthony Campbell knew that acupuncture worked, and wrote books on their interpretation and its use, but they grappled with the concepts of TCM. A lot of research has been done since then, and is still ongoing

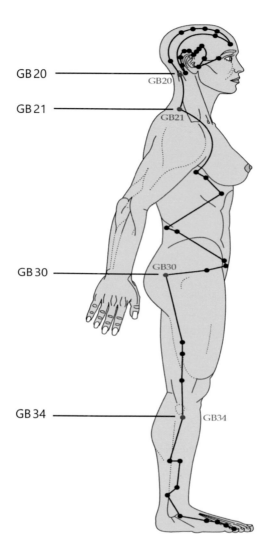

GB 20

GB 21

GB 30

GB 34

Fig. 1: The Gall Bladder (GB) channel showing four commonly used points.
Courtesy of Dr Mike Cummings.

thanks to scientists like the Swedish physiologist Thomas Lundeberg, who is trying to understand its complex neurophysiological basis. When it comes to reducing pain, it is well known that acupuncture stimulates specific nerve fibres to the spinal cord, and these inhibit onward passage of pain impulses to the brain and also stimulate release of opiates. Approaches to treatment can vary as well as the choice of points. TCM points can be used, that are known to have specific effects, such as PC6 (point number 6 on the Pericardium Channel) on the inside of the wrist, which is useful for treating nausea and vomiting. Segmental points affect nerves from the spinal cord that supply a specific area of pain. Trigger points are painful fingertip-sized areas found in a taut band of muscle, which can cause chronic pain and stiffness. Many of them correlate with traditional acupuncture points. Some practitioners may needle trigger points only, and this technique may be referred to as 'dry needling' instead of acupuncture.

Much of what I learnt about trigger points seemed to fit in with my massage knowledge – the loosening of taut bands and identifying particularly tender spots – but I hadn't heard the phrase 'trigger points'. The work of the American doctor, Janet Travell, which began in the 1950s, has been significant for understanding trigger points and the common patterns of pain associated with them. She realised that whichever hospital ward she worked on, many patients were in pain that was often unrelated to their condition. Their muscles were not routinely examined, but when she did so, she found many pain points. Travell and Simons wrote a two-volume book called *Myofascial Pain and Dysfunction: The Trigger Point Manual*. It was published first in 1983, and again in 1998, and it has been the standard text for trigger-point treatment since being updated into a single volume by an editorial board (published in 2013). The word 'myofascial' relates to muscles (myo) and the layers of connective tissue (fascia); they enclose muscles and separate them into layers. The term 'myofascial syndrome' was coined to describe the associated muscle pain.

In that first course, I was taught about some of the common patterns of pain distribution in the body, depending on the muscle involved, and trained to treat a select number of points on the upper and lower body. By understanding these patterns and points, acupuncture could be used to treat chronic pain and musculoskeletal disorders, particularly back pain and migraine (even if no particular muscular tension is identified).

Debates were raging throughout medical establishments in the UK and elsewhere about the effectiveness of acupuncture. How much could be put down to the placebo effect ('all in the mind'), how should trials be conducted, how much it should be used alongside as an alternative to conventional treatments? I decided I needed to know what acupuncture felt like, and to feel its effects for myself.

Reactions to acupuncture with needles

I felt nervous when the time came to practise on each other, and although we had all been thoroughly briefed, Mandy looked even more nervous than me. It isn't ideal to practise on someone who doesn't need treatment, but the experience of needle placement and what insertion feels like gives invaluable insights and understanding about your own and others' reactions to needling. Mandy volunteered to be the first 'patient' in our group. I held back to watch the others do it first. Once seated, Mandy had a needle inserted into the thick trapezius muscle between her shoulder and neck (the thick pinchable one at the base of the neck), at the point GB21 (as shown in Fig. 1).

I watched her muscle being grasped between the student's thumb and fingers as it was lifted up and pulled away from her chest wall, to make sure the needle went nowhere near the pleural cavity that houses the lungs. If a needle penetrates this cavity, air can become trapped inside and cause a lung to collapse. Although we all had medical knowledge, we had to revise the important anatomical areas and which features to avoid. Rare though complications are in acupuncture, they can happen. Certain muscles can develop something called compartment syndrome, whereby a needle causes bleeding and pressure builds up, potentially compressing a nerve fibre or blood vessel. Bleeding can also happen if a needle penetrates a joint space – or the needle could break. Varicose veins must be avoided, too, because they can be so easily damaged.

This is why the training was so important, to minimise such risks, to make sure we understood the anatomy and practised safely. It also highlighted the importance of knowing a client's medical history and about any current medical treatment. For example, blood pressure can drop during acupuncture, so clients who already have low blood pressure can faint. And it cannot be performed on a client who is taking the blood thinner warfarin following a thrombosis (blood clot), unless their warfarin levels are well controlled.

Unexpected reactions can happen too, but Mandy's reaction that day certainly got everyone's attention. Within a couple of minutes of the needle being placed in her shoulder she said, in a quiet voice, 'Look at this'. She held out both her hands, palms facing upwards. Droplets of sweat covered the one on her left – there were none on the right. And she told us she didn't feel well. The needle was quickly removed and she recovered quickly. That was the first of many memorable lessons about acupuncture needles, and the powerful effects brought about by stimulating the nerves and muscles in the body.

The course also included a demonstration of electro-acupuncture. This is where two needles are inserted at sites up to a few inches apart in an area chosen for stimulation, and connected to a power pack. This is a stronger form of acupuncture, often used now to treat osteoarthritis of the knees by passing a current across the joint. I volunteered to be treated this way and watched one needle being place in the web of my thumb and the other just below my elbow. The needles caused a slight ache, which didn't bother me, but as soon as the power was turned on, a strong pain surged up my arm.

"That's *de Qi*," Jonny the supervising doctor explained, referring to the boost of energy sometimes felt with needle stimulation. But it felt exactly like the shock I received on holiday near Aviemore, where as a teenager for some strange reason, I knowingly touched an electric fence surrounding a warthog pen at what is now called the Highland Wildlife Park.

I was convinced it was an electric shock I had felt and was disappointed that it wasn't *de Qi*. Jonny didn't use the machine again that day, but a few days later he confirmed that the machine had short-circuited and indeed I had been shocked from its battery. He said it was a training session he wouldn't forget!

It took several years for me to get back into electro-acupuncture. I attended a course and began, tentatively at first, to use the new machine I was provided with. Now I use the technique regularly for treating chronic pain, and do so with total confidence thanks to my much more advanced machine! My husband Kenneth was probably the first patient I treated and to this day he loves to get electro-acupuncture whenever he has any inkling of back pain (although he sometimes complains he would be treated more quickly if he booked an appointment with me through official channels!).

A touch of homeopathy

I wasn't going to be at Carol's practice long enough to be able to offer consecutive weeks of acupuncture treatment to our cat and dog patients, but she was keen for me to treat her own dog, Guy. His hind limbs were stiffening up. When she witnessed the improvement, she went on to train in acupuncture too, making it a regular part of her practice.

She was happy for me to advise on homeopathy, though, which I did for a few cases. It astounded me that when a German Shepherd stopped being car sick after receiving *Argentum nitricum* before travelling. Later, in another practice, I used *Symphytum officianale*, nicknamed 'knit-bone', from the Comfrey plant. I tried this treatment on a dog and a cat who were heading for leg amputations because of broken bones that hadn't united properly; both of them recovered and their legs were functional again – albeit slightly squint.

One day, a colleague of mine phoned me up after seeing a hamster with a fractured foreleg a week after I'd prescribed a daily *Symphytum* tablet in its drinking water. She wanted to know what treatment I had given it, because the limb had healed so well. I remember being told on the course I'd attended that the undetectable changes to the water molecules are like those in two DVDs that have identical chemical components yet they play different movies. However, I didn't pursue homeopathy any further than that, not least because of the lack of scientific evidence for it, which means there is still great scepticism about its use in medicine. Saying that, I still use *Arnica* for bruising and wounds, and two veterinary classmates of mine went on to train in homeopathy and consider it useful in small-animal practice.

Veterinary acupuncture in Wiltshire (November 1999)

Wiltshire is not an easy place to get to from Fife, but that's where I headed for my next course. Everyone else on the course was a beginner in the field of veterinary acupuncture. We were told that only vets were allowed to treat animals using acupuncture but, in fact, it has since been clarified that trained veterinary nurses under veterinary supervision can do so too. We were reminded how safe it was and how well animals tolerated it. The main reasons for using it with animals were pretty much the same as those for using it with humans, namely to avoid side effects from conventional medicines, allowing use of a lower dose (or perhaps none at all); or because the options from conventional medicine had been exhausted; or because the cost of other treatment was prohibitive. It could be used alongside conventional treatment, hence it was complementary. What it wasn't, however, was a cure-all.

The course was based on traditional Chinese medicine, in which emotional, hereditary and environmental influences are believed to produce a particular disease pattern. Acupuncture is thought to restore equilibrium between the physical, emotional and spiritual aspects of the body, correcting any imbalances in Yin and Yang, and aiming to improve flow of the vital energy Qi (also spelt Chi) and 'blood' (not the same as 'blood' in western medicine).

We were told it was likely that acupuncture developed from acupressure – a needle-less technique based on the same principles – and was used when some vet schools were first established until acupuncture was superseded by newer treatments. It was explained that acupuncture was supported by advances in scientific knowledge and had been widely accepted since the 1970s, not least because science can explain many of the effects of acupuncture (although not all of them) and reputable journals such as *Pain* publish articles on it.

The Yin and Yang of traditional Chinese medicine equate to the two arms of the autonomic nervous system – the parasympathetic (for resting, digesting and repairing) and the sympathetic (for fight or flight) – and its automatic or subconscious effects. Acupuncture has an effect on these, as well as the hypothalamus, a regulation centre in the brain that has links to the pituitary gland, which is why it works on internal medical disorders. However, it is known to be most effective for chronic disorders and pain.

The channels are fundamental to traditional Chinese medicine, but their existence is disputed in Western medicine, which more often relies on anatomical knowledge and clinical experience for point selection. We learned some basics of the traditional form, and about point location, and how to insert and manipulate needles, and how points on the human body could be translocated to animals with some minor alterations due to anatomical variations. I learned that acupuncture could also do a lot more than just treat pain.

At the end of the course, I had seen several dogs and horses being treated for a variety of conditions, mostly to do with mobility and sore backs and joints. They were accustomed to acupuncture and quite accepting of it, absolutely relaxed about it despite the number of students gathering around them. The atmosphere was always calm. Sometimes the needles were taken out straight away, or left in place for anywhere from a few minutes to twenty minutes, always depending on the type of animal, its particular needs and its response.

I was beginning to feel more in tune with acupuncture, but I felt even more encouraged after meeting vet Ann Hutchison of Dalblair Veterinary Surgery in Ayr at a talk she gave.

As well as being qualified in homeopathy, Ann had an international qualification in acupuncture and used it regularly to treat small animals and horses. She was so committed to it that she had started on a degree course in traditional Chinese acupuncture at Reading University. She said that it gave her a different approach to and interpretation of health and disease, as well as adding to her understanding of how the body works.

I was lucky because she offered to give me advice and help at any time – I just had to get started! But it would be another year before that opportunity arose.

The millennium

I worked Mondays to Fridays in a mixed practice, leaving my weekends free for taking courses. I saw pets in the clinic, but didn't have enough large-animal experience to be on-call for the local farmers seven days a week. I was happy with this – the odd horse or cow visits I'd helped with had been nerve-racking!

Some evenings, I crossed the river from Fife to the Edinburgh side, and noticed the numbers on the overhead signs of the brightly lit Forth Bridge counting down towards the millennium. The close of the twentieth century was a time of great anticipation and heralded many changes ahead for me.

More locum work followed in Dunfermline and Kirkcaldy. I even found myself back in Australia for a couple of months, in Adelaide, South Australia, and back on-call to help out at a friend's practice. I was still resolved not to get tied down to my own small-animal practice, despite being drawn to clinical work. I would have to be on-call again – so hard after a busy day in the clinic, and it was impossible to relax. Starting a permanent full-time job and being on-call again was going to be a challenge.

Carol used an external company to provide emergency cover, which is commonplace nowadays. She defended her decision strongly to a client of hers who complained about how impersonal it was, telling them how many vets faced mental health problems because of the workload, and how they have a higher-than-average suicide rate. If it helped take the pressure off her staff, Carol thought, then it was well worth doing.

Of course, I did want to settle down, somewhere and sometime in the future. And I hoped to incorporate acupuncture into my veterinary work. That conference in Tasmania had been a turning point in my career, but far more momentous than that was re-meeting one of my old school friends when I returned home in 1999 – and, in 2002, becoming a wife to Kenneth and a step-mum to Pamela and Kirk!

— 3 —
Early cases

*Why does watching a dog be a dog fill one
with happiness?*
Jonathan Safran, American novelist

By August 2000, I was back in full-time practice with Ryan and Calder in Dunfermline (now Albavet). My bosses, Joe and Aileen, were happy for me to use my acupuncture skills. While it felt exciting to be introducing a different type of treatment, I needed to be convinced that acupuncture would work for me. I had many questions. Would it really make a difference? Would all the animals allow me to do it, or only some? Would the owners be interested in trying it or was it simply just too 'whacky'? And would I actually have time for it if it was indeed accepted? Appointments were fitted in between operations and routine consultations, and interest amongst staff and clients was slowly to gather momentum.

I explained to clients that some conditions take five to twelve treatments, but four were more common, given once a week or fortnightly – a more realistic commitment. I assured them that if no benefit was detected, treatment would be discontinued. For acute problems such as muscle strain, one treatment or a short course might resolve the condition but chronic ones including arthritis would need follow-up or top-up treatments every few weeks, aiming to increase the intervals between sessions. If given too frequently, the pet's body can become used to the stimulation and therefore less responsive.

As explained previously, there are variations in point selection, the size and length of the needles and the time they are left in for. There are points on the ears that can be used, but I have never done this on animals – humans, yes – but needles would fly everywhere if a dog or cat shook their head and, worse still, they might disappear down the ear canal! In those early days, I didn't use electro-acupuncture for the more chronic conditions, let alone laser acupuncture, which is brilliant for more sensitive cases.

The most common requests were for help with pain and mobility and to avoid drug side effects. Doctors and vets are lucky to have a wide choice of painkillers to prescribe for their patients now. Years ago, steroids were often used for anti-inflammatory treatment and animal painkillers were virtually non-existent. Different 'families' of drugs work in different ways, and a variety are available on prescription nowadays, with similar ones for use in animals, some for acute pain and others for chronic pain, which persists for three months or more. The choice of drug also depends on the severity of pain to be targeted – mild or moderate or severe. Pain also has different origins; it might be neuropathic, meaning it is affected by the nervous system, so a drug like gabapentin may be prescribed.

Vets must adhere to what is known as the 'cascade' protocol, first using drugs that are licensed for animals, and then off-licence drugs (only for human use) but only if the options run out. Off-licence drugs haven't been tested in animals (just humans) but they are considered safe enough. They include amitriptyline, amantadine and gabapentin, and the owner's permission is needed up front. The opiate tramadol used to fall into this category but is now licensed for dogs and cats.

The dose of drug depends on the animal's weight, and that needs to be measured accurately to avoid toxicity. Drug interactions are a concern, too, which can happen when more than one type of drug is given at a time. There are also some differences between species on how drugs are metabolised. For example, aspirin is toxic to cats because they lack the enzyme needed to degrade it, and paracetamol can be toxic to dogs.

Meloxicam is a non-steroidal anti-inflammatory drug (NSAID for short) and a common first-choice of painkiller for dogs and cats – and humans, although we humans tend to use similar non-prescription ones like ibuprofen. It can be very effective at reducing pain, but they have to be used safely and an eye kept out for possible side effects, such as lethargy, loss of appetite, vomiting, diarrhoea and blood loss. In extreme cases, kidney failure may occur, even death. Similarly, tramadol can cause lethargy, sedation, vomiting and constipation (which is more likely than diarrhoea).

The effectiveness, or efficacy, of a drug in any animal can't be known without trying it out, and some owners are reluctant to use them, preferring 'natural' remedies. There's a huge array of non-prescription remedies (which are still medicines) on-line, such as turmeric and various cannabis-based preparations, but there is little evidence that they are effective. This isn't to say they don't work, but without undergoing proper trials, under well-controlled conditions, neither vets (nor doctors) can readily recommend them. The most important factor of all, in all types of medicine, is to do no harm. Here I describe some of the acupuncture cases I saw over the early years. It didn't take me long to be convinced of its value!

Oscar and Ishka—two black Labradors

My first patient was Oscar the dog, a Labrador, and Pat was his owner. The veterinary nurse Yvonne had suggested she tried acupuncture. She and all the other staff in the practice had been on the lookout for suitable cases and Oscar seemed ideal. He had been diagnosed with hip dysplasia at a young age, before Pat had got him from a rescue home. This is where the ball and socket of the hip joint do not form properly, so the hips can be misshapen. A more extreme case is shown in the x-ray below.

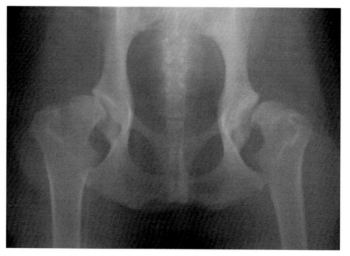

An x-ray of hip dysplasia in a dog, showing the lack of proper ball and socket joints.

Understandably, it can cause a lot of discomfort and can progress to arthritis. Often there is a hereditary component, more common among certain breeds, so dams and sires are usually screened and given a hip-score, then only the low scorers are used for breeding. Even so, this doesn't guarantee that the pups will be trouble free.

At nine years of age, Oscar had bouts of stiffness in his back legs. Pat brought him in for courses of anti-inflammatory injections or tablets but felt these weren't working as well as before. She wanted to see what acupuncture could do for him.

Oscar loved coming to the practice, always happy and full of beans. Nothing fazed him. The problem was keeping him in one place so I could insert the needles. Getting him onto the consulting table was bit of a pantomime, so we tried it on the floor. Unlike human patients, he danced around the room and kept fidgeting! In the end, he did settle down, sitting on the floor with Pat beside him, giving him a good cuddle. He was fine when I treated his back and hind legs, but when I inserted a needle at a point in his knee, he jumped up sharply, with a fleeting 'Ouch.' This is a strong balancing point, according to Chinese medicine, and Oscar often reacted to it – but then forgot about it just as quickly.

After only two treatments, Pat noticed that Oscar was livelier and could jump into the car more easily. Over the following months, he only needed top-ups every few weeks. Then he went lame on one of his front legs, and his elbows felt enlarged. I did an x-ray and found that he had osteoarthritis in his elbows too. I kept going with acupuncture and put him on another anti-inflammatory drug. But he went off his food and had a stomach upset. Blood tests showed his liver enzymes were raised, so I had to stop the painkiller and treat his liver.

He continued to get acupuncture every few weeks and managed just fine for another two years until he was almost twelve, when the liver problem overtook him. You will hear more about him in Chapter 11.

Pat had another black Lab, Ishka, also with mobility problems, but unfortunately acupuncture wasn't going to help her. She received a course of acupuncture when she became a little lame, but the lameness became severe. X-rays showed she had severe spinal spondylosis, where bony spurs grow out across the gap between the spinal vertebrae, restricting movements and causing neuromuscular pain. The nerve supply to Ishka's leg was affected and nothing more could be done for her – painkillers were of no help.

This shows that while acupuncture has a role in many conditions, including spondylosis, there are times when it is not appropriate. And if it is not helping, other solutions are needed, which may mean putting to sleep.

Scamp—the Heinz 57 mongrel

I told owners that their pets would probably be relaxed and sleepy after a treatment, but for Scamp, a Heinz-variety type of dog, this was not the case. After his first treatment he went home and tried to mount Elizabeth's other dog, Lady, despite being neutered. His mobility had improved greatly, so much so, in fact, that the *Sunday Post* became interested and the three of us featured in an article on animal acupuncture.

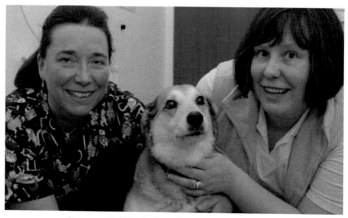

Scamp with Elizabeth and me in The Sunday Post.

Scamp was especially memorable because he allowed himself to be treated for another condition that Elizabeth and I wouldn't have wanted for ourselves! This was a large cyst-type growth on his eyelid; it was unsightly and it was beginning to bother him. I wondered whether he would cope with needles placed in his eyelid in an attempt to shrink it, and I told Elizabeth the story of Blue, in Tasmania, who had sat completely still as I removed the piece of grass lodged across his eye.

Like Blue, Scamp just sat there as I started the Chinese technique known as circling the dragon. It involves inserting needles in a circle, as close to the damaged skin as possible.

Some days later, Scamp's cyst burst and shrank considerably. It didn't completely disappear, but he no longer needed surgery to remove it. After that, I found many other uses for circling the dragon, which is why I have dedicated a whole chapter to the subject (see Chapter 11).

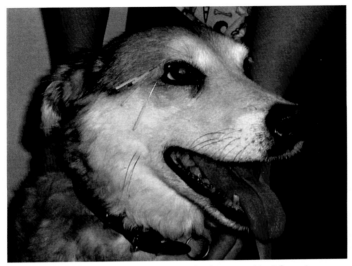

Scamp unbothered by me circling the dragon on his right eye!

I have often felt very humbled by the trust animals put in us, and my experiences with Blue and Scamp are up there at the top.

Buster the Cavalier

Most of my acupuncture cases were elderly and large-breed dogs. Buster was different. He was only two years old and a Cavalier King Charles Spaniel. According to his owner, Margaret, he had become reluctant to walk very far and seemed to be stiff. His spine had been x-rayed previously, and when nothing was found he was sent to a specialist orthopaedic vet.

Further x-rays revealed he had hip dysplasia, like Oscar, which is not at all common in Cavaliers and surprised us all at the practice. Buster would sit placidly on the examination table as I used similar points to

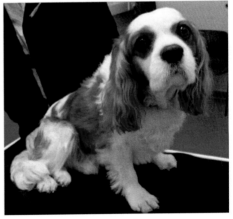

A young Buster – coming for acupuncture when he couldn't jump on the bed!

those I used with Oscar, often eliciting twitches along his back where his muscles had tightened.

Not only did acupuncture keep Buster mobile, but he could also jump onto the bed again. Margaret only needed to bring him in for top-ups when he stopped being able to do this. He didn't need painkillers for many years, not until his arthritis eventually progressed, but it was his breed tendency for heart failure that let him down in the end.

Griff and Grace—the Springers

Springer Spaniels Griff and Grace were also early cases. Griff came first because he had a 'lick' granuloma, a bald area of skin caused by constant licking – quite a common problem in dogs. Antibiotics can help to fight infections if the skin gets broken, and anti-inflammatories can help, but often the licking starts again. Griff didn't mind me circling the dragon at all. After one session, he left the area alone and never bothered with it again.

Owners Malcolm and Lindsay were regulars at the practice – and I knew Griff's insides intimately! He was a scavenger and had to be operated on several times to remove foreign bodies that he'd swallowed and had got stuck in his intestines – causing a blockage and causing him to be miserable and not eating, not passing any stools and vomiting. On one occasion it was a piece of corn on the cob. He was so crafty that even with a muzzle on he could find a way to eat things that he shouldn't have. This time, he was brought in for obvious musculo-skeletal pain. He had lumbar spondylosis and arthritis in his wrist (carpal) joints. He didn't tolerate anti-

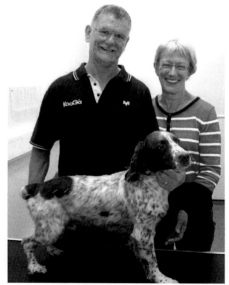

Griff, the scavenger, who lived to 15! (with owners Malcolm and Lindsay.)

inflammatories so for four years I gave him acupuncture regularly. He did well and, despite everything, lived to the grand age of fifteen.

Sometimes Grace came along for acupuncture too, as she also had hip dysplasia. Like Griff, her mobility was helped massively by her slimness.

Gromit, another of Malcolm and Lindsay's Springers, is pictured with Grace below. They are sitting in front of a health-advisory poster on the wall, but they didn't need their weight checked!

It may seem obvious, but if sore joints have less weight to carry then not being overweight is a huge help – it's the same for animals and humans although it is often overlooked! There is more about the significance of weight in Chapter 13.

I often found that when one pet in a family began to get acupuncture, the treatment was readily accepted by their owners, often leading to a succession of pets coming in for similar treatment over the years, and allowing me to get to know them really well.

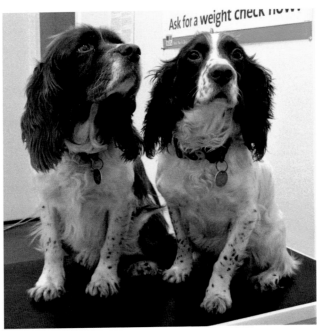

Gromit and Grace – always slim, which
helped with their mobility.

Lewis and Harris—Newfoundland giants

My vet colleague Rachel was always very open to trying acupuncture for different conditions and Lewis's case sounded intriguing because it had an easily measurable target – his coat. His mobility was affected by spinal and hip arthritis, and it had improved with medication alone, but his coat was threadbare, with many bald patches, possibly as a side effect of his tablets. The question was posed by Rachel – could we use acupuncture to maintain his mobility, reduce his medication and see if his hair grew back? I thought about Ishka and her severe spondylosis, which acupuncture hadn't been appropriate for, but knew Lewis had nothing like her level of symptoms. Being a Newfoundland, and weighing in at around fifty-five kilos, he was one of the biggest dogs I have ever treated.

It felt exciting. Lewis's vet and his owners were willing to try it out, but what about Lewis himself? How would such a powerful dog react? His owner John said he thought Lewis would be okay – luckily his other dog, Harris, didn't need any treatment. He would be another kettle of fish entirely, John told me.

The acupuncture certainly helped Lewis's mobility, and his medication was reduced from six tablets a day of prednoleucotropin (abbreviated to PLT; it includes the drugs cinchophen and prednisolone) to one a day, thus getting rid of the side effects and allowing his fur to regrow. John chose not to give up on Lewis's medication entirely.

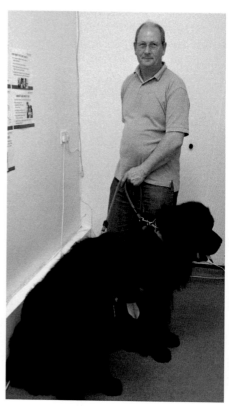

With owner John - Harris and Lewis, both weighing in at at least 55 kilograms.

He kept going with the one-sixth dose (which would have had a minuscule pain-relieving effect), but I could see how Lewis moved and responded to joint manipulation and everyone enjoyed his lush new coat. It's worth saying that even with monthly acupuncture treatment, this regimen was more cost effective for the insurance company.

Lewis's response was truly satisfying. To my ever-present naysayer mind, this was very strong evidence of the effectiveness of acupuncture. One of the problems about it being accepted into mainstream medicine is getting 'proof' in the clinical-trial context; such studies are plagued by a lack of funding, or inappropriate design of the experiments, or difficult-to-measure outcomes.

A couple of years later it was Harris's turn, when his mobility worsened. Remembering John's words, I was a little nervous, but Harris surprised both of us – it was a big relief to see he was as laid-back as Lewis about the acupuncture.

It wasn't just creaky hips he was contending with, though. He also had ataxia, due to a failing nerve supply to the legs, which made him unsteady. Instead of his back legs moving separately they would crossover as he pirouetted to turn a corner. He often had a wide-based stance as he tried not to wobble, making him look drunk.

I also went on to use electro-acupuncture to treat him, one of the first cases I used it in, ensuring he got extra stimulation from the electric current passing between two needles.

John still talks about how much acupuncture improved the quality of life for both his dogs, and alleviated their need for more medication. They both lived to the age of twelve, which is pretty exceptional for such a large breed.

I had the pleasure of showing Lewis off at one of my acupuncture talks. My husband Kenneth remembers how impressive it was when a huge Lewis lumbered into the venue and quietly laid in front of the audience throughout his treatment.

Compliance with treatment – Izzy and other dogs

Some dogs are very wary when they visit the vets, and may even tremble during the examination. Spaniel Izzy is one such dog. She still hides beneath her owner's seat in the waiting room, although now she is braver, brave enough even to snaffle down a treat after her acupuncture session! Izzy is pictured *overpage*.

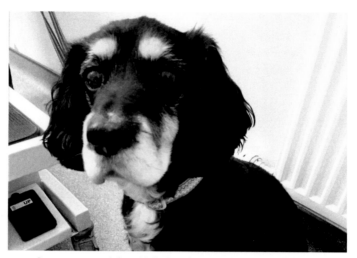

Izzy comes round the table looking for a treat after acupuncture!

I have found that other dogs that were previously averse to coming to the vets, become excited and happy to come in once they have had acupuncture, sometimes straining at the lead to come into the consulting room.

Kola the Labrador took her time. Owner Alison knew just how nervous Kola got that she asked the nurse, Helaina, who knew Kola outside work, to accompany them to Kola's first acupuncture session for her lameness. Alison was delighted when Kola settled down and became more comfortable – even more so, when, after just a few sessions, she sauntered happily into the clinic.

Spending a long time in the consulting room can be stressful for some pets. Vets work around this in different ways, but I found that appointments of thirty to forty-five minutes for a first assessment with treatment and further sessions of twenty to thirty minutes work fine, but some degree of flexibility is always needed! For dogs like Kola, it is best to keep treatments short until their confidence grows. For some, it makes no difference, especially with suspicious cats!

Ben the Golden Retriever had to be coaxed out of the car into the waiting room, then led to the consulting room in stages, with treats along the way. It was his first visit to the practice, and he was suspicious; he seemed to sense it was a vets. At eleven years old, he was streetwise! His owner Kristeen was worried how he would take

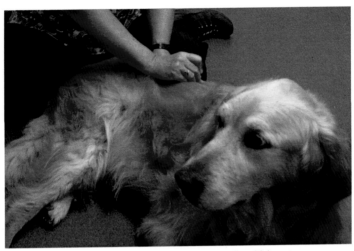

*Ben overcame his initial reluctance and couldn't wait
to get into the acupuncture room!*

to acupuncture, but after a few sessions he was eager to come into the building. He came straight up to the door of my room and lay down on the floor outside it, waiting for his turn. His sore hips soon improved and Kristeen was delighted.

I am humbled by Kristeen's interpretation, opinions and her words. When I contacted her about her and Ben's experiences (this was five years after Ben died), she sent me this letter:

Ben, our adorable Golden Retriever, began to show signs of sore hips around the age of 9 or 10 and started off with Metacam, which helped for a while. As the disease progressed he moved onto stronger medication, such as Tramadol and PLT, which we gradually increased until he was taking over twenty tablets a day. He was such a biddable boy; he'd open his mouth for me and swallow them, knowing a gravy bone or two would come afterwards.

One morning, as I was popping these pills down his throat, I couldn't help but think that surely there must be another way; I hated doing this to him. Would I want to be taking twenty tablets a day? The tablets had also given him ulcers so he was having an upset stomach on a regular basis. I decided enough was enough. I had to find another way to help him, or face that dreaded decision of 'doing the right thing.' So I started searching the internet and came across various articles on alternative medicines, acupuncture being one of them.

The next day I saw my vet and asked if acupuncture was something we could explore. I'd known it to help some of my human friends with back pain and suchlike, so might it help my furry one? My vet told me about Jane Hunter, a vet who now devoted her career to acupuncture, and that some of his patients had had a degree of success with it. So an appointment was set up and the following week I took Ben to see her.

Ben was very tentative at first, needing to be coaxed in the door, but he soon knew this was different. Jane got down on the floor with him, stroked his head and talked to him. Then she inserted the needles around his body, from his neck to his toes, behind his ears and along his back. He rarely ever flinched. At the end, a treat was dispensed and off he went, feeling very relaxed. He enjoyed a good snooze in the boot on the way home.

Sessions were weekly for the first month and I began to detect a change in him. He was definitely moving better and keener to walk a little further than before. We were onto something here - we now had a plan for the long term for Ben. He loved his sessions with Jane so much that as we entered the surgery, I'd take off his lead and he'd wander straight up to her door and lie there, paws crossed, waiting for her. He genuinely liked coming to see her. I have no doubt Ben knew it was good for him. After each session, Jane would decide if we could start dropping some of the opiates he was on, and gradually, over time, Ben was taking only one tablet a day, from over twenty tablets when she first started working with him. Sessions would be fortnightly, but sometimes they'd be spaced out a little further, depending on how well he was moving.

Ben's life changed thanks to Jane and her skill. He enjoyed his walks and was able to walk further than he had done in a long time. Most pleasing of all, he regained his spark, which had been snuffed out by the medication he'd been on. We continued with his acupuncture up until he died, at the age of 13 (which was unrelated to his arthritis). It was undoubtedly one of the best things I ever did for him and he enjoyed another two years of happy, quality living. A pragmatic piece of advice I would give to any pet owner is to consider choosing a pet insurance plan that covers alternative therapies.

I am a great advocate of acupuncture and have recommended it to others. I carry a picture on my phone of Ben receiving his treatment from Jane and show it to people who are in a dilemma about what to do with their poorly pet when conventional medicine no longer works. Acupuncture will always be in our medicine cupboard, and it has proven to me that there are different ways - other than pills - that can do as good, if not better, at managing pain and other ailments.

It's true that owners can be overly optimistic at the start of treatment, sometimes believing things have improved permanently after one or two treatments, but if the improvement isn't genuine then it doesn't last. This is why a minimum of four sessions are given, on average, to allow the pet to be observed and assessed over time; it is sometimes life-changing, as with Ben. Having used acupuncture for more than twenty years, my naysayer voice reminds me that I still need to be convinced by positive changes, despite the fact that most cases are like Sasha, with her spinal spondylosis, whose new lease of life was witnessed by her owner and me, and her eagerness to visit me for treatments never abated.

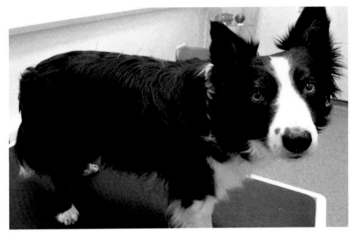

Sasha with needles along her spine – always keen to come in for acupuncture!

The safety aspects of acupuncture

In the consulting room, safety is paramount for all animals, owners and vets. I have heard of many events and stories from general practice, so I know that very unexpected things can happen from time to time. There have been reports of animals not being held properly by their owners and falling off the consulting table, resulting in a broken leg and heated debate over who should pay the bill!

In reality it can be hard to stay alert for everything that might happen. One of my colleagues had a nasty bite from a dog that wasn't being examined – it was just watching its friend being checked over on the table, presumably trying to protect it. I've experienced a few surprises of my own. One particularly hot day, one of my clients was accompanied by a friend, who stood quietly at the back of the consulting room, before slumping to the floor in a pile. We had no idea there was anything amiss until she fainted. On another occasion, I felt very uncomfortable when a client assured me it was fine to empty the anal glands of her huge Great Dane with her toddler loose in the room. It wasn't just the contents of the 'rear end' I was worried about, but if the child was near the 'head end' the dog could bite as a reflex to my actions. Thankfully, neither end caused any trouble and the toddler left intact and unstained!

Acupuncture consultations are no different, but fortunately there have only been a handful of dogs I haven't been able to treat. I remember one Weimaraner and one Labrador, both so hyper that they wouldn't stay still long enough for me to place a needle, so I had to stop trying. The Labrador, even when high up on the table, would jump vertically, making treatment impossible. Because we are aiming to encourage relaxation I always feel that for acupuncture it is best not to restrain an animal by anything more than a cuddle. If that fails, then best left alone.

Two dogs I tried to treat simply had a nasty streak, and weren't worth risking a finger for. Sometimes a muzzle can be used to ensure both the vet and owner's safety. Another two dogs were so unpredictable that their owners were very worried about how they would react, so it wasn't appropriate to try and treat them. Some dogs, like Nell and Sisko, had huge reactions to needling, which I will come to later, in Chapter 9.

Another safety issue with acupuncture is making sure that needles don't get lost, not just down an ear canal or after being shaken across the room, but keeping track of them in the pile of a fur coat (a major difference between treating a person and an animal!). Needless to say (no pun intended!), needles always need to be counted in and counted out.

Assessing the effects of acupuncture

The effects of acupuncture on an animal vary so much that it all comes down to assessment on a case-by-case basis. There can be visible improvements if lameness decreases or resolves, or if the animal reacts less to palpation and joint manipulation (indicating that they are in less pain), but only the owners can observe their pets' behavioural changes in the home and the outdoors. German Shepherd Meg had

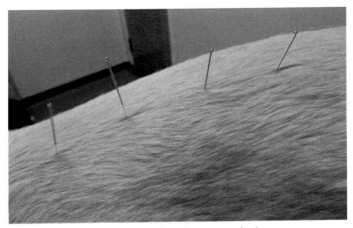

Needles nicely visible in the fur coat of a dog.

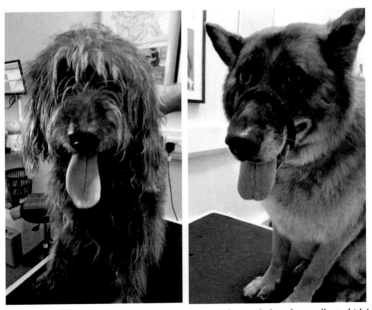

Ness and Danny – the shaggiest, thickest of coats and a good place for needles to hide!

acupuncture with unusual results. The first thing her owner said on arriving for their appointment after a few treatments was, 'What a night I've had!'. I thought she meant that Meg had been unwell. Vomiting and diarrhoea, perhaps? But that wasn't it. Left in the house alone, Meg had completely destroyed her bed, leaving stuffing and torn fabric all over the place. Oh dear, I thought. But Meg's owner was actually delighted! Meg had felt so good after acupuncture that she was behaving normally (albeit badly) again!

More often than not, acupuncture has a calming effect, but another helpful side effect was noticed by Max's owner. Max the Old English Sheepdog could be grumpy with other dogs in the park, but once he started having acupuncture for forelimb lameness he began behaving much better and was far less worrisome. We concluded that acupuncture was helping Max's forelimb; he was in less discomfort and more relaxed overall, so generally less irritable!

Changes such as those displayed by Meg and Max are difficult to record in a suitable format for providing scientific evidence. There are methods for 'scoring' pain, as there are for humans, produced by university researchers, which change over the years and are especially useful for hospital patients. When it comes to veterinary practice, however, in addition to examination we still mostly rely on the owners' interpretations, thus I have always worked by identifying the key problems and recording any observed changes.

More recently there has been a push towards the use of 'stance-analyser' platforms. These record the way the animal's weight is distributed on each limb, and any pressure changes, so they enable the degree of lameness to be measured. Changes can be noted and no doubt will be of more use in the future in measuring the success of treatments.

Meanwhile, after spending three years of using acupuncture to treat pets – mostly dogs (only a few cats, though, which have their own chapter) – I was absolutely convinced of its value in veterinary medicine. However, shockingly and unbelievably I lost both of my parents in May 2002 and after struggling on for a year or so I knew I had to take a break from full-time work. And I found I had some decisions to make ...

— 4 —
Can you treat me too?

Leaving my full-time position at Ryan and Calder meant there would be no one to continue treating the regular acupuncture cases. Their needs could be met, however, if I worked just one day a week. So Thursday became my acupuncture day. Instead of fitting cases in between routine consultations or operating duties, I would have the luxury of time and be able to focus entirely on acupuncture.

I had learned how versatile acupuncture could be for animals and what an impact it could have. I could treat the young and the old, with or without medication alongside, and I knew there was a certain place for it in veterinary practice alongside conventional treatment.

I greatly appreciated how flexible and supportive the practice had been about me establishing a standalone acupuncture clinic. However, it was when I was treating Oscar one day that Pat looked me straight in the eye with a quizzical, earnest face and asked, "Can you treat me?".

I felt something fundamental shift inside me. Having completed both massage and acupuncture courses for people, I had a never-ending supply of volunteers among my family, friends and work colleagues who were happy to be 'guinea pigs', but I'd never had the time to take it further.

Pat was so impressed by what acupuncture had done for Oscar that she wanted to try it for herself. She suffered from polymyalgia, meaning she had muscular pains in multiple parts of her body, and she had always relied on steroids to help her. She did whatever else she could to help herself, keeping active by walking her three dogs and attending Pilates classes.

I wondered if acupuncture could help her, but said she would need to ask her doctor first whether it was available on the NHS. If not, would I be allowed to treat her, given that I was a vet? My mind was swimming with the possibilities.

The room felt peaceful that day. It was quiet in the practice, with no extraneous barking or commotion. Oscar was settled on the floor, lying on his side, with the needle hubs visible above his fur, completely oblivious to the significance of that conversation between Pat and me.

Millhill GP surgery, March 2004—a new beginning

While I felt a strong connection with massage and working with people, I hadn't counted on acupuncture coming into the equation. After a great deal of discussion with my husband Kenneth, and him expressing his unwavering support, it felt right to explore my options. I was able to get the relevant complementary-health insurance and decided it would be ideal to offer acupuncture from my own premises, but I couldn't commit to renting somewhere for an untried venture. I kept putting off looking up doctors' surgeries in the Yellow Pages because I felt embarrassed – a vet phoning a GP practice to ask to rent a room to do acupuncture in felt a bit odd!

I started by phoning the closest practice to our house. The first call was met with a simple answer – no spare room here! The second said something similar, but also told me not to mention Reiki, in which I was also trained – a hands-on Japanese healing technique, where, in theory, energy flow in the body contributes to wellbeing, It is classed as an alternative therapy and regarded by many scientists as pseudo-science. Acupuncture and massage seemed to be acceptable. I felt slightly more optimistic at this point – it didn't seem such an outlandish request after all. And when I called the third practice, I struck gold. I was told, 'Yes. There is a room, depending on the day of the week you need it. Would you like to visit on Monday?'.

Monday morning came quickly and everything was perfectly straightforward. It was a lovely big room, and I could use it for two afternoons a week, and pay monthly. Did I have a letter of introduction? It was happening so fast. No, I didn't have a letter with me but I told the receptionist I would be back shortly. That lunchtime I searched through pile after pile of boxes in the garage for the last CV I'd written, dating from some four years previously. I could use it for my professional history with a covering letter to describe more recent events, together with a request to the GPs to rent the room. So, two weeks later in March 2004 – five months after leaving full-time veterinary work – I was starting a new job. At least, I hoped I was. It all depended on people booking appointments to see me.

I felt nervous and excited on my first day at Millhill and was quite overcome when the receptionist handed me a beautiful bouquet of flowers. Scamp's owner, Elizabeth, had very thoughtfully had them delivered, to wish me luck. Elizabeth and Pat had been among my first (human) patients. Little did I know then that I would be working successfully at Millhill for the next sixteen years, progressing to the use of laser and electro-acupuncture, or that GP Liz would become such a close friend, and one day get me on a road bike!

During that first year, the momentum grew steadily, largely by word of mouth. Because I was working privately, I couldn't advertise my clinics for people within the NHS surgery, but I could at the veterinary clinic. The appointments lasted from thirty to sixty minutes, depending on the treatment I was carrying out. My two afternoons at the surgery finished at six in the evening, when the surgery closed, but I also sometimes worked until as late as nine at the vets on a Thursday – treating people. They were mostly existing clients of the vet practice, who were pleased to be able to come after work and weren't fazed whatsoever about using the operating table in the theatre – conveniently it was a human one, acquired from a local hospital. The room was kitted out with the same hygienic standards as the GP surgery, with sharps and waste-disposal facilities, and there was no problem when Fife Council instigated the new licensing rules for acupuncture premises. The late appointment times were very popular and my clients often enjoyed the hilarity it caused when they told their friends they were going to the vets – for treatment for themselves!

My human-patient caseload and experience duly built up alongside the veterinary, but I was very conscious that I was a vet treating people. While having a degree in traditional Chinese acupuncture would be the icing on the cake, I felt I couldn't justify another three years of expensive study to learn a completely different approach, given that I was able to practice with the qualifications I already had.

However, I did make sure I attended BMAS training days and meetings, aware that once I had enough cases under my belt I could then do their Certificate. And there was a massive bonus – Liz was one of the senior GPs and already a BMAS member and trained. She had already treated a few of her patients but her time was very restricted. I will be forever indebted to her for the additional medical advice she gave me, and of course her friendship.

Acupuncture certification—2005

I was at a BMAS conference, listening to someone describe what was involved in obtaining their further qualifications. The Certificate of

Basic Competence (COBC) was the first step, so I worked towards having thirty cases and attending the required number of courses. The COBC is now called the Certificate in Medical Acupuncture (CMA).

On the day of the practical exam in Glasgow, Pat was a willing accomplice as my sample patient. I struggled to contain my laughter when the examiner turned around and saw Pat stripped to her underwear! She didn't need to reveal quite so much for the purposes of the exam, but that was Pat's wholehearted style.

After completing the COBC in 2005, I sighed to myself when I realised I couldn't stop there. There was also a Diploma I felt I needed to have, although it was at a different level altogether. It involved one hundred hours of training and writing up fifteen cases, all in great depth and all on different topics. Not many of us went on to complete the Diploma and, at that point, no vets had. I would be breaking new ground, which made me a bit anxious, but I felt if I didn't do it soon then I never would. I was very lucky to be based in the GP surgery and could run my ideas by Liz. Within my two years of treating people, I already had a range of interesting cases.

What yoga has done for me

At around this time my interest in yoga was developing. Ever since going to classes taught by my schoolfriend Ian, when I was twenty-three years old, I attended a yoga class no matter where I lived. Yoga may look relaxed and easy to observers, but it isn't easy, and it has always made me aware of how much more flexible I could be. It has always been important to me to work within my own limits, and to avoid injury through overstretching or overextending, even when tempted to keep up with those around me! The relaxation period, sometimes meditation, is always a joy, but fitting in plenty of good poses and stretches is what keeps me going. Ian's classes were hard to beat – we held poses for a long time, and afterwards I could feel my muscles ache.

Ian is a remarkable person. He had a serious car accident in which he broke several bones in his legs and had to be cut from the wreckage. Before the emergency team arrived, he pushed himself up with one hand on the glass-less window and the other on the back of the seat, holding the position so as to realign his broken bones as best he could, working with his breath just to stay conscious.

"Call it instinct?" he told me. "But I remember strongly thinking – if

I pass out, it's curtains. I obviously had a very raised awareness due to the endorphin rush and I think the yoga training held it all together."

Ian soon had everyone on his ward doing yoga with him, including breathing exercises and meditation. He also astounded the surgeons with his recovery.

While yoga has come in and out of my life, I found it comforting to attend classes at a local gym when I lost my parents. The bereavement had been tough. In 2004 the teacher was also involved in running a course for aspiring yoga teachers. With only two places left, I sent in my application so fast that the passport photo I included was taken after rushing out from the swimming pool, my still-wet hair plastered to my head. Kenneth couldn't believe I was prepared to submit such an awful photo – I even had it on my passport for the next ten years!

The yoga course ran while I was still building up my cases for the COBC and Diploma, and I could see how all the threads of my training were coming together.

In short, I could use massage to palpate and identify problem areas at the same time as loosening muscles; I could use acupuncture to work on trigger points and stimulate nerves and muscles at a deeper level; and I could recommend yoga exercises or a class for patients to loosen and relax.

Something I learned quite quickly is how much our repetitive habits contribute to strains and injuries. Our bodies are not designed to sit for hours in the same position, whether working at a computer, driving without a break or lounging on a sofa. There are different ways to describe ailments like this, like repetitive strain injury (RSI) or, as they say in New Zealand, occupational overuse syndrome (OOS), which is linked specifically to a job.

In New Zealand, my friend Sheryll was diagnosed with OOS and pain in her shoulder linked to her office job, whereby she had to set an alarm at the other side of the room and get up from her seat to switch it off every fifteen minutes.

However, prevention is always better than cure, which is why trying to avoid repetitive actions is vital, and fitting in some regular stretching, whether through yoga, Pilates or physiotherapy, is so important.

Diploma in Medical Acupuncture—2006

By 2006, the new professional role I had built up was really exciting. I was self-employed and back doing veterinary locum work, while running an acupuncture clinic for dogs and cats at Ryan and Calder's practice; I had extended my clinic hours for people at the GP surgery and was running a weekly yoga class as a qualified teacher. With all of this going on, it took considerable effort to stay focused on fulfilling the requirements of the Diploma.

I was very lucky to have Liz and also Jack, another GP in the practice, to look over my in-depth written cases, and I could also refer to my allocated GP mentor Val, who had already completed her BMAS Diploma. She advised me to send in seventeen cases instead of the required fifteen, just in case any failed. And so it was that in May 2006, after just over two years of treating people and having sat a practical exam, I breathed a huge sigh of relief when I was awarded my Diploma – official proof that as a vet I was also trained to treat people. The studying continues. To maintain my BMAS accreditation, I need to do six hours continuing professional development (CPD) every year, and another thirty-five to meet veterinary requirements.

There has always been plenty of variety in my work, but it was all possible because of the similarities between humans and animals. Animals are so like humans that all human analgesics have been developed and tested on animal models. And determining the level of pain an animal is experiencing is as difficult as it is for doctors when dealing with young children who don't communicate verbally.

Ian Self, a veterinary specialist in anaesthesia and analgesia, reminds us that 'if it hurts us, it will hurt them' (our animals).

The similarities don't end there. When I was explaining the problems our cat Guinness was having to my nephew Ross, then a medical student, he was amazed to hear that cats have a thyroid gland just the same as humans!

All you have to do is compare the skeletons of a human and a dog, as shown on the opposite page. The bones have pretty much the same names, although the human knee joint is called the stifle in a dog, and the ankle is the hock (tarsus).

The spine is arranged the same way, too, with similar numbering of the spinal vertebrae (see the table *overpage*).

OPPOSITE: The skeletons of a human (Fig. 2 top) and a dog (Fig. 3 bottom). Note the similarities between them, particularly the structure of the spine, with its cervical, thoracic and lumbar vertebrae, and the pelvis, sacrum and coccyx. Images courtesy of Alexander Pokusay@adobestock and magicmine@adobestock.

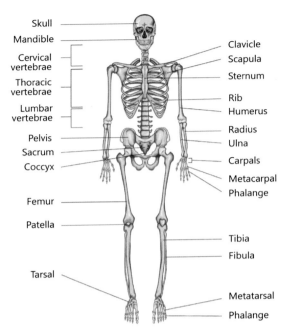

Skull
Mandible
Cervical vertebrae
Thoracic vertebrae
Lumbar vertebrae
Pelvis
Sacrum
Coccyx
Femur
Patella
Tarsal

Clavicle
Scapula
Sternum
Rib
Humerus
Radius
Ulna
Carpals
Metacarpal
Phalange
Tibia
Fibula
Metatarsal
Phalange

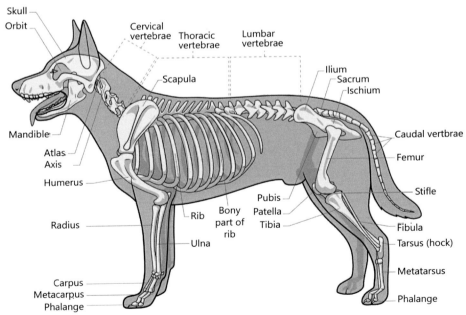

Skull
Orbit
Cervical vertebrae
Thoracic vertebrae
Lumbar vertebrae
Scapula
Ilium
Sacrum
Ischium
Mandible
Atlas
Axis
Humerus
Caudal vertbrae
Femur
Radius
Stifle
Pubis
Patella
Tibia
Rib
Bony part of rib
Fibula
Tarsus (hock)
Ulna
Metatarsus
Carpus
Metacarpus
Phalange
Phalange

Spinal region	Name of vertebrae	In humans	In dogs/cats
Neck	Cervical (C)	7 (C1–C7)	7 (C1–C7)
Cervicothoracic (CT) relating to neck/chest region			
Chest	Thoracic (T)	12 (T1–T12)	13 (T1–T13)
Thoracolumbar (TL) relating to chest/lower back region			
Lower back	Lumbar (L)	5 (L1–L5)	7 (L1–L7)
Lumbosacral (LS) relating to lower back/pelvic region			
Pelvis	Sacral (S)	5 (fused)	3 (fused)
Sacrococcygeal (SCo) relating to pelvic/coccyx region			
Coccyx or tail	Coccygeal (Co) or caudal	3–5 (fused)	6–23+ (depends on breed)

The names and numbers of spinal vertebrae and regions in humans, dogs and cats.

The people I treated while preparing for my Diploma had many different disorders including back pain (e.g. sciatica), osteoarthritis of the hip and knee, rotator cuff tendinitis (a shoulder problem), golfer's elbow, neck pain, headaches and migraine, irritable bowel syndrome (IBS), fibromyalgia and piriformis syndrome (more on this in Chapter 7).

I also saw some unusual cases, including someone with kaleidoscopic vision. I will tell you about some of these in the following chapters – along with tales relating to dogs and cats.

— 5 —
The shoulders and above

The National Institute for Health and Care Excellence (NICE) provides numerous guidelines for NHS England and Wales on the best treatment options for specific conditions. These guidelines are also used by NHS Scotland who, in addition, have their own, referred to as SIGN (Scottish Intercollegiate Guidelines Network).

The NICE *Management of Headaches* document of 2018 advises using aspirin, paracetamol or an NSAID for acute treatment of tension-type headaches (TTH), and the option of a course of up to ten sessions of acupuncture over five to eight weeks for migraines and tension-related headaches. Of note there is no mention at all of acupuncture for any condition in the SIGN guidelines.

Three of the cases that I submitted for my Diploma were linked with migraine, headaches and shoulder tension and all of them were significant for different reasons. While tension-related headaches and migraines can be well-defined as separate conditions, there is quite a lot of overlap.

Treating sceptical Bryan's neck pain and headaches

In my experience, while medical professionals advise on treatment for others they often avoid or postpone their own, and are generally the last to seek help for themselves! I knew that my dentist brother-in-law, Bryan, was very sceptical about acupuncture and was only trying it because he was desperate! He had taken time off work due to tonsillitis and frequent headaches up the back and left side of his head, for which he was taking Syndol™, a mix of paracetamol, caffeine, codeine and doxylamine. He had coped with frequent headaches, neck pain and stiffness and occasional migraines for twenty years by then (for the site of his head pain, see Fig. 4 *overpage*).

Three years before talking to me, he experienced numbness in the fourth and fifth fingers of his left hand and the outside of his arm. An x-ray revealed some arthritic changes to his cervical vertebrae with narrowed disc space between C5 and C6. This was partly attributed to normal 'wear and tear' and his occupation. Bryan took ibuprofen for the pain and received physiotherapy until the neurological symptoms eventually went away.

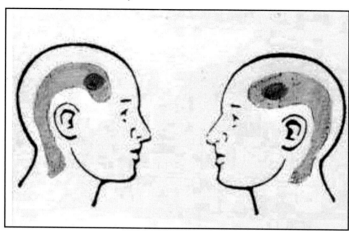

Fig. 4: A map of Bryan's head pain (both sides). Hand-drawn by the author.

■ Major pain

■ Minor pain

At 46 years of age, Bryan found his job increasingly demanding and was aware that he felt very tense on workdays. The forty-five-minute drive each way didn't help. The tension was especially bad when he went back to work after a weekend or holiday. Although he was aware of correct body posture, the tension in his neck and shoulders built up during the day, after hours of bending over dental chair. He had tension headaches at least once a week, and (but only rarely) migraines. He kept himself fit by exercising regularly and running and windsurfing.

When I examined him, he had no pain or tightness at his shoulder joints, but he had restricted rotation of his neck in both directions, especially to the left side. What was very obvious to me, as he lay down on his front for treatment, were two identical raised taut bands around 10 cm long that ran from each upper free border of his trapezius muscles at the base of his neck, down to the angle of his shoulder blades (Fig. 5). Both of these bands were extremely painful to the touch, and had apparent trigger points in the upper, middle and lower parts. The base of the left band felt 'gristlier' than that on the right (see triangles on the map). There was some tension in his neck muscles, but no trigger points, so the bands were the most significant finding.

According to two textbooks I had been reading at the time, by Baldry and Gunn, the pattern of Bryan's pain was typical of the Travell and Simons' map of the area where muscle tension leads to tension headaches. He was a textbook case!

A visual analogue score (VAS) is a simple pain-scoring system in which the patient marks on a 10-cm horizontal line an estimation of their pain, where the left of the line signifies no pain (0), and the right of the line signifies maximum pain (100). Bryan registered 64 out of 100. The bands were so obvious and so painful to touch that, assuming he would need some follow-up sessions, I decided to treat the trigger points alone to gauge an initial response. The upper point corresponded to GB21 (Fig. 1), which is a well-known point for helping with neck pain and headaches. I inserted three needles at these points as shown by the triangles within the taut bands in Fig. 5.

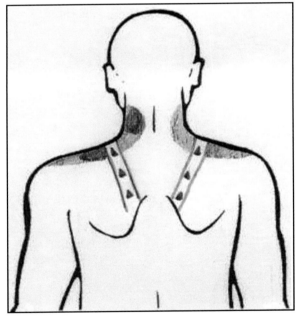

Fig. 5: A map of Bryan's neck and shoulder pain. Hand-drawn by the author.

■ Major pain

■ Minor pain

▲ Trigger points

Stripes = taut bands

At the second session, one week later, Bryan's pain score had reduced to 25 out of 100 and his neck movement was much improved. The taut band on the left was no longer palpable (able to be felt) and the one on the right had shortened by half, to just five centimetres. He hadn't had any more headaches. Based on this, I needled GB21 (Fig. 1) on both sides and also below the right trapezius band.

Both of the taut bands had gone by the third session. Bryan was aware of only slight tension in his neck and upper shoulders. He did so well that he didn't need another session for two months when the tension had built up again.

Bryan's case clearly demonstrated the immense value of acupuncture for managing chronic muscle tension and its knock-on effects, even with a very sceptical patient like Bryan! He never suffered such a bad bout of pain again, or felt the need for more acupuncture because of his work. Attending a regular Pilates class helped him too, but the very best thing he did for himself was to retire!

Lynsey's migraines

It was obvious with Bryan's job that all that bending over patients would put a huge strain on the muscles between his shoulders and the base of his skull (the occipital area). But sitting at a computer all day long was the contributing factor for Lynsey. Her job in the oil industry was very stressful, with long hours and always chasing a deadline. She had been plagued by headaches and migraines for three months, sometimes having to take days off. The area of pain she described is shown in Fig. 6 – it was different from Bryan's. At just thirty-one years old she was one of my youngest patients but she'd been diagnosed with migraine at the age of twenty-one, when she had been studying away from home. Her doctor had prescribed daily pizotifen on two occasions over the years, which had been effective, but Lynsey wanted to see what acupuncture could do for her, in the hope of avoiding more medication.

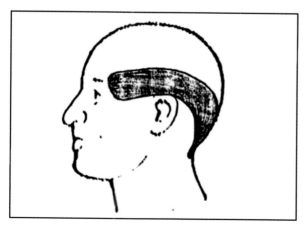

Fig. 6: A map of Lynsey's head pain. Hand-drawn by the author.

She told me she had some tension in her shoulders and neck. On massage, some of her muscles were taut and painful but there were no obvious trigger points. I suspected they lay deeper than I could get to because she was too sore for firmer pressure. So I tried a combination of local acupuncture points and the ones on the hands and feet that are recommended for migraine – a combination of distal acupuncture points and ones where there are usually trigger points.

Because of work commitments, Lynsey could only come and see me once a month, for a total of three treatments, because she was moving abroad. She said, "The relief I got from acupuncture from the headaches helped me think more clearly and therefore I could reassess my job and lifestyle and make changes". Life did indeed change; a new job eventually led to meeting her partner and starting a family!

Neil's visual disturbance

Bryan and Lynsey were typical of the human cases I saw over the next fifteen years, but I have never had another case like Neil's. He came to me after having disturbed vision for two whole weeks. There was no pain but he could see coloured spots, as if he were looking through a kaleidoscope. His GP suspected an unusual type of migraine (scintillating scotoma) and signed him off from work as a sound engineer. Neil had been prone to migraines every few months since he was eight years old, but then, at the age of twenty-three, he was finding it very different and scary. He was miserable, stuck at home and couldn't even read or watch television.

While I knew there could be very serious causes for his symptoms, he had been examined recently by his doctor. Despite feeling the head pain and nausea often associated with migraine, the unusual visual symptoms were still thought to be migraine-related, and they hadn't worsened. His doctor thought acupuncture would be worth trying. Neil wasn't sleeping well, and felt tired all the time. Sometimes his arms went numb. His usual Migraleve™ tablets (a combination of buclizine, paracetamol and codeine) were having no effect.

He was certainly looking pale and tired when I first saw him, and my heart sank when he described his routine. He worked twelve-hour shifts or longer, sitting in a windowless room, usually with tight deadlines to meet. He had no time for exercise, he told me, and had given up playing football. His diet wasn't healthy and he could easily smoke up to twenty cigarettes a day.

I felt hesitant about treating Neil because of his unusual symptoms, but an appointment with a neurologist was in the pipeline. His usual symptoms were headache and nausea, occasionally vomiting, but the visual disturbance was new for him, and something that both he and his parents were particularly anxious about. His parents, who he lived with, even considered cancelling their imminent holiday to Australia, so time was of the essence. We all felt there was a chance acupuncture could help, and it was well worth trying. There was nothing to lose, and everything to gain.

I arranged to treat him once or twice a week, depending on his reaction. Neil was actually wondering if the problem could be related to having previously taken maximum doses of paracetamol for a bad toothache, which had been followed by a migraine.

To my surprise, when I began to examine and massage his shoulder and neck muscles, there was no increased tension. In fact, quite the opposite – there was very little muscle tone; not a taut band or trigger point in sight. This was very different from other cases of migraine and tension-type headaches I'd worked with before, so I concentrated on using the points recommended for migraine in the foot, hand, neck and shoulder. There was a visible twitch when I put a needle in his foot, which was a sure sign that the acupuncture was having an effect.

At the second treatment, just two days later, Neil reported that the visual spots were the same but he had a good night's sleep and felt better in himself. After eight days he came for his third treatment, after which he said he had fewer spots and for two days had felt the best he had done for quite a while. However, a visit to the dentist for fillings resulted in two bad days. By the time I saw him again, the spots had worsened and he had a headache for which he had taken ibuprofen. I included some extra acupuncture points this time, but Neil felt one was uncomfortable and another one was itchy, so I stopped using them.

A week later I gave him his fourth treatment. He was still off work and wasn't taking any medication. His doctor had referred him to the migraine clinic at the hospital as well as an optical specialist, and recommended that he continued with the acupuncture while he was waiting. Neil was feeling much better in himself, though, and generally functioning and sleeping better, although still seeing some dots. The toothache was gone completely and he described a feeling of pressure, rather than pain, in his head. His vision had improved slightly and he could read and watch television again, although this made the coloured spots more noticeable.

He saw the specialist who identified migraine as the cause and prescribed valproate medication, which is usually prescribed as an anti-epileptic and is unlicensed for the treatment of migraine. The specialist explained that lifestyle factors were a major contributor and that addressing these issues was really important. Slowly Neil improved and was able to return to work after a month, even though his vision was not completely normal. But after several months, it disappeared and to the best of my knowledge did not return.

It was an unusual symptom and I was delighted to help him. Resting from his normal routine, plus a new medication and acupuncture no doubt all contributed in some measure. Neil certainly felt that acupuncture helped him cope with his symptoms, possibly caused them to lessen somewhat, at a time when he felt at least something had to be done.

There is another migraine sufferer who stands out in my memory because of the severity of his symptoms. David was a GP and very keen to try acupuncture – and there was a measurable response.

Dr David's cervical spondylosis

Cervical spondylosis had been diagnosed on an x-ray and David had pretty much accepted the best option for him was pain medication. He didn't think anything else would make a difference. However, he was regularly getting severe pain at the back of his head, around the bony lump at the base of his skull (in the occipital area), which could lead to a migraine and this really worried him.

Spondylosis can develop at any level of the spine in both humans and animals, but cervical spondylosis affects the neck. It is common in people aged forty onwards. Just as in animals, bony spurs (osteophytes) can develop between the vertebrae, causing restricted movement and neuromuscular pain and, if a nerve gets trapped, the pain can be severe and affect the arms.

A GP colleague at David's practice had already been to me for back treatment and urged David to give acupuncture a go. After a headache that lasted ten long days – and with his wife nagging him to do something about it – David eventually gave in and made an appointment with the vet!

He categorised his symptoms into three areas – recurring migraines, occipital pain and arthritis in his neck. A migraine could develop following tension in his shoulders, especially on the right side, but at other times there was no known trigger as far as he was aware. He could go for weeks without a migraine and then have several in the space of a few days. Sometimes he had pins and needles in his arms, most often when he woke up in the morning. This was from the nerve involvement. Anti-inflammatories and paracetamol didn't give him much relief, but he did take migraine medication sometimes. Much of what he was describing sounded like Bryan, so I showed him the map of Bryan's pain and areas where I used needles to treat him. David was surprised to see how similar the highlighted areas were to his own areas of pain.

I explained what I was planning to do in more detail than usual and then started to massage him. The trapezius muscles across the top of his shoulders were like bricks, and I hadn't even reached his neck. The muscle tension was incredible, all across his shoulder blades, especially the rhomboids near the spine, and running up the sides of his neck. His right side was more sensitive and there was a very gristly band of muscle between the base of his neck and his shoulder blade. I soon had to ease off because just a little extra pressure made David very sore. He had never had a deep-tissue massage before and he was astounded by what he was feeling. His muscles relaxed a little and I could pinpoint his trigger points – fingertip-sized areas that produced exquisite pain when pressed.

I warned David that he might have an almighty headache that night. The treatment was new to him and if he was sensitive to it, it could make things worse before they got better. That night he did indeed have a bad migraine, but the following morning, the pain at the back of his head had virtually disappeared! He came for several more treatments over the subsequent weeks, encouraged because of the reduction in his headaches. After three months, he told me he hadn't had any bad ones since the first session. His pain score had gone from 75 out of 100 to zero.

David said he had underestimated the significance of muscle tension, and had instead put his pain down to the arthritic changes in his neck. This persuaded him that massage and acupuncture was a powerful combination. He improved so much that he eventually stopped coming for regular treatment, popping back every few months or so when he decided he needed a refresh. He also found ways to manage better by doing yoga, specifically arm, neck and shoulder stretches, which he could fit in at any time of day (but he said he felt a bit self-conscious doing them when he was walking down the street!).

When Eileen came for a top-up treatment in early 2019, I had a draft version of David's story in my bag. I had pulled the notes out of my shoebox filing system (it worked well enough for me from the start) the evening before, and was planning to write his story up, after not looking at his or the other stories I'd collated for years. I had recently talked to his wife, Joyce, who gave me permission to include his case in this book. He had died more than seven years previously. We reminisced about him, and how massage and acupuncture had been the only treatment that gave him proper relief from his headaches.

So, I was totally taken aback when out of the blue Eileen began talking about 'Dr David' – the one and the same – several years after his death and on the very day I just so happened to have his notes with me. It was uncanny! Eileen was speaking about him, very fondly, about what an excellent GP he had been and how he was one of the loveliest people she knew.

I had known Eileen for quite a long time. Her husband William had complained of a sore shoulder and been to see his GP – who was, of course, Dr David. Part of William's problem was long-distance driving, plus an awkward heavy manual job and the fact that he wasn't getting any younger. Dr David thought the soreness was mostly muscular and he was concerned that William might have to wait for several weeks before seeing an NHS physiotherapist. So (while he admitted that he shouldn't be doing so), he suggested to William that he should seek help privately. He gave him my name. This suited William very well, especially because he could visit me at a time that coincided with his shifts.

He came for several massage treatments that eased his shoulder and kept him functioning at work until he retired. Sometimes Eileen was our go-between on the phone, and it was really good to finally meet her, some years later, when she needed help with sciatica. She too had been recommended by her GP to have massage privately because the physiotherapy list was three months long at that point. Eileen had remembered me because of her husband, which led to this amazing coincidence.

Her walking was a little improved by the time she came to see me but she had been frightened by the severity of the sciatic pain and how debilitating it was. For her, the regular massage and acupuncture treatments helped to keep the pain at bay. She was doing very well at helping herself, by keeping up her walking and using a static exercise bike, but one day she dismounted it awkwardly and felt something 'go'. We worked out she must have lifted her right leg a bit higher than usual, but we were back to square one. This time she was panicking – in a few weeks she was due to travel to America with William on a special trip.

I'm pleased to say that with weekly treatment Eileen recovered – just in time for their holiday – and I felt relieved to see her go in much better shape. I just hoped she would remain free from pain – the long flight would be quite a challenge. The next I heard from her was when I received postcard from New York with the simple message, 'Thank you!'

A note on dogs and headaches

I've been asked a few times "Do dogs get headaches?". Obviously there is no clear answer to this – but it's unlikely to occur often because they don't have the same mechanics or lifestyle habits as people. But they may get headaches if there is some underlying condition or disease.

It can be difficult to know if acupuncture has helped a patient, whether dog or person, but I do know that even when their symptoms persist they can become less anxious and therefore cope better. No doubt even the feeling that 'something is being done' can be helpful in humans, perhaps a placebo effect, but I don't think this is true for animals!

The next two canine cases are a good example of the difference acupuncture can make, even from the sceptical owners' point of view!

—6—
'New' backs for old dogs!

As 2007 rolled in, I had a new opportunity to do two mornings a week as a veterinary locum at the Glenrothes branch of the St Clair Veterinary Group. John, one of the partners, had finally decided to retire (completely) and I was asked to fill the gap.

It felt like I had been full circle. I'd been to the practice at its old premises in Commercial Street in Kirkcaldy when I was still at school. Back then, it was known as Smith and Boyd, a mixed practice treating cattle, sheep and horses, but with an increasing volume of small-animal work.

When the careers-guidance teacher at Beath High school asked me what I wanted to study, I plucked up the courage and told her I was thinking of applying for veterinary medicine. She looked horrified! "Being a vet is a man's job," she snapped. "What about nursing administration?". Luckily, another one of my teachers was not horrified at all. He was a friend of John at Smith and Boyd.

I usually did my work experience after school and was fortunate to meet a wide variety of owners with their dogs, cats and occasionally 'others'. The clinics seemed to go on forever. There were no appointments and no computers; and it was pot-luck who would turn up, and how many of them. At least it gave me some idea of how hectic a vet's schedule could be, and some of the positives and negatives of practice. It took quite an effort to catch the two buses back home to Cowdenbeath from Kirkcaldy, especially on the cold winter nights, but while watching animals be put to sleep was sad, it was to end suffering, and nothing I saw in the clinic put me off.

I can still remember John giving me a blunt talking to, saying that if I felt at all unwell while watching an operation I was to leave the room. I never expected to have any problems but when the first large German Shepherd I saw lay on the table, mid-spay with its innards on show, it happened. Spots appeared in my vision as my hearing faded, and just in time I remembered John's instruction to leave the room. I made a beeline for the door, but luckily I didn't pass out. And I have never felt like that again.

The St Clair clinic I returned to was a far cry from the 1970's version. It had a purpose-built hospital and far more staff. It even went on to win a national veterinary-clinic award in 2009. Coincidentally, John had introduced acupuncture to the practice, which I was able to continue (although I could never fill his shoes). The number of cases built up slowly as the partners came to appreciate the difference acupuncture made to some of the animals they referred. When the treatments began taking up too much of my consulting time, around 2010, the idea of setting up a separate acupuncture clinic was supported, meaning that I could see more cases by extending my working week. It was at this time that Oz the dog was referred to me.

A new lease of life for Oz

Oz's lovely whiskery Spaniel face looked worried, yet he stood quietly on the table after being reluctantly lifted onto it. His owner explained she had brought him to me after Jarlath, one of the partners, had recommended acupuncture for Oz. Various medications had been tried on Oz, but he was still miserable. Acupuncture was a last resort, and literally the end of the road for him.

He was not yet ten years old but he had shown signs of back pain and stiffness for a while. Jarlath had spoken to me about him and explained that his owners, Christine and her husband Ed, believed his quality of life was so poor that they were considering putting him to sleep out of kindness.

As it turned out, they were also sceptical about acupuncture. They had no expectations, but simply decided to follow Jarlath's advice because it was the last option. Christine felt that if he recommended it then it was within veterinary regulations, and as it was to be performed by someone who was qualified and had a good track record, then they had nothing to lose. After thirty years in jewellery retail management, travelling all over Scotland, Christine had taken early retirement to spend more time with Oz, and her husband Ed who had his own health issues. They wanted to do all they could for Oz, and had even moved house to accommodate his mobility problems.

I found on studying Oz's medical history that the main reasons for considering acupuncture were his poor mobility and weakness in his right hind leg. Recent x-rays of his spine and hips showed severe spondylosis, the same as in Dr David's neck. There were ridges of bone where there should be spaces between the vertebrae of his lumbar spine, and he had marked osteoarthritis in both hip joints. The joints had far less range of motion than a normal ball-and-socket joint and his back had lost its flexibility, resulting in pain and stiffness. Acupuncture couldn't help with the bony changes but it might help release the tight painful muscles around Oz's affected joints and stimulate useful anti-inflammatory reactions and natural-opiate (endorphin) release from his brain. I just wanted to help him … if he would let me.

But Oz had a chequered past! There was a long list of incidents in his ten-year life, stretching back to when he was a pup. He had a gastrointestinal upset when he was only a few weeks old; the diarrhoea went on for days, and he underwent many investigations. His surgical wound, following routine castration, became infected and needed antibiotics. Later he choked on a stick and collapsed, but thankfully it was removed promptly enough by an on-duty nurse at the practice. At the age of four he began to stagger about, and was put onto lifelong treatment for epilepsy. On another occasion he ate a full net bag of bird food and had to be admitted for induced vomiting – he was a dreadful thief (although I never saw that side of him; he looked very innocent!).

Christine says she will never forget the day of Oz's first acupuncture session as long as she lives. She had no idea what it entailed and was worried how Oz would be; she knew that if he was frightened, he might bite. We were careful that she had a firm hold of him, with her arm around his neck, while I inserted a needle at a sedation point at the back of his head before working along his back. What she didn't

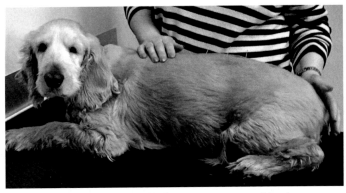

Oz chilled out on the table during acupuncture to his spine.

expect was him to nearly fall asleep in her arms, his head heavy on her arm as she supported his weight. More pleasing than that, even, she saw an immediate difference in his demeanour. Straight after his treatment he wanted to go for a walk – something he hadn't shown interest in for quite a while.

Christine and Ed were nothing short of amazed. Oz returned to his previous boisterous self after just a few treatments. Jarlath was pleased too, and relieved to see the improvement that acupuncture had brought about. As for me, I was happy it had been such a positive experience for Oz and his owners.

True to form, Oz had yet more ups and downs (luckily minor ones) over the next four years, involving regular trips to the vets for various issues. It was suspected that he had Cushing's disease but the test results were inconclusive. One time he stole and ate a half pound of butter, another time he had a sinus (a type of abscess) on his foot; large warts grew that had to be surgically removed under anaesthetic, but he recovered well. His fur thinned out too, but that improved with thyroid medication. As time went by he needed more help with his pain, for which he received meloxicam or tramadol alongside his acupuncture.

Then life finally caught up with Oz. He became quite vocal and restless, possibly due to some form of dementia and his health was generally failing. Jarlath put him to sleep at the age of thirteen. Christine maintains that she and Ed had all these extra years with Oz because of the fantastic results he had with acupuncture. For both her and Ed, he had been living proof of its effectiveness.

Acupuncture led to another problem for Buddy's owner!

Buddy's owner, Candy, was also very sceptical about alternative therapies, but there was no predicting how acupuncture was going to change Buddy's life! In 2006, Buddy was seven years old. A Lhasa Apso with attitude. Candy warned me, "He can bite!". It seemed hard to believe as I tousled the hair on his cute fluffy face, but I did know he had a powerful set of teeth. This was the first time I met Buddy and I wondered how he would cope with acupuncture. Buddy had been struggling with back pain for some time, and Candy had been surprised when acupuncture had been recommended by her regular vet. She admitted she felt nervous and doubted whether he would go along with it – he was a feisty character!

Over the previous two years, Buddy's episodes of severe lumbar pain had reoccurred every three or four months and needed anti-inflammatory medication. Ten months before coming to my clinic, there was nothing significant on his x-rays, nor were there any clinical signs of the nerves to his hind legs being affected. The next step would be referral to a specialist for a myelogram, in which a contrast dye is injected into the spinal canal to reveal any narrowing, where a disc may be pressing on a nerve, but Candy was hoping to avoid all that that entailed. At least Buddy would respond with rest and an anti-inflammatory called Rimadyl™. His last painful bout had been a month before and since then things had settled, but Candy felt he was often lethargic, and just miserable. The big question was, could acupuncture stop these bouts of pain returning and let Buddy lead a more normal life? Four acupuncture sessions were planned – if this was acceptable to Buddy of course.

Candy didn't want to use a muzzle so she tried holding his nose, despite the fact that it was so short and didn't offer much to grip. Often there is a trade-off between upsetting a dog by using a muzzle but being safe oneself, and going along with the owner's wishes. I sensed Buddy was going to be tricky. He had the cutest face, but there was a glint in his eye and he was very suspicious. I trusted Candy, though, and said we'd give it a go without the muzzle.

I began with a needle into a superficial calming point at the back of the head, then gingerly inserted more needles at the master point for arthritis, between the shoulder blades. All the needles were inserted superficially only because this was his first time. He was doing better than I had expected, but Candy and I both stayed on high alert. I should point out that my reflexes are sometimes embarrassingly quick – an animal can sneeze and I've already jumped out of the way, but it's amazing how quickly dogs can turn to bite. As I worked on points away from his back, Buddy flinched a little at a point on his knee. And when I reached the taut muscles of his lumbar spine he growled and turned around at a needle on his left side. But that was as far as he went. He had done very well for his first session. At later sessions, Candy and I never knew when he was going to react, but he would react every time. He always had something to say!

Buddy was sleepy for two days following that first session, and Candy noticed that he was lying in more stretched out and relaxed

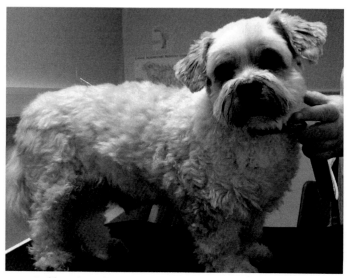

Buddy with needles showing on his spine – sweet looking but feisty!

positions. At his second treatment a week later, his back muscles felt less taut to me. He yawned with the relaxing effect of the needling and sat well through the session, but the points on his back remained sensitive, with lots of twitching going on. Overall, though, he showed signs of being very responsive to the treatment. Candy relaxed too when Buddy was sleepy.

When she brought Buddy in for his third treatment she looked crestfallen. I assumed the worst – that he had relapsed – but he was moving briskly along the corridor, looking positively perky. And that was the problem, it seems. Buddy was now too perky! His medication had been stopped and he was exercising more, but this included being sexually active again, and he had started mounting everything and anything – a human leg or anything soft and fluffy! I couldn't help laughing, but Candy struggled to see the funny side. It was a sure sign Buddy's back had improved; he could stand on his hind legs again, and he was obviously more flexible! But Candy was upset because she had been advised to have him neutered. I had to agree that it was the best long-term solution. It wasn't what Candy wanted to hear, but his behaviour was problematic.

This sexual hyperactivity after acupuncture was new to me, and it made me wonder whether Buddy had always been in some degree of pain, which had inhibited his mounting behaviour. Male dogs usually start to mount at only a few months old, which is why neutering is often carried out then. Although Candy was delighted to see the change in Buddy's life overall, the thought of him going through a general anaesthetic and surgery worried her. I tried to reassure her that removing his testicles would have several health benefits, as well as stopping him mounting; it would prevent his prostate from becoming enlarged and making it difficult to go the toilet; it would prevent anal adenomas (growths that are influenced by testosterone); and it would prevent testicular tumours from forming.

Candy was still worried, however, but she arranged the operation. Buddy sailed through with no problem and after a few weeks, when his testosterone levels fell, he stopped mounting. Furthermore, the muscles in his back had softened and he no longer needed anti-inflammatories. Candy was enjoying her much easier life with Buddy, especially because he was far less aggressive when he sat at the living-room window to watch passers-by. He was happier too about being picked up and was, in general, much more agreeable and settled.

After only seven acupuncture treatments, delivered over four months, Buddy's top-ups were spaced out to every two or three months. He was on his best behaviour when he came along with Candy to a talk I was giving, and sat quietly on a seat next to her as I presented his case to the audience.

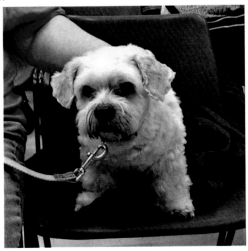

Buddy 'listening' at one of my talks.

Buddy did so well, in fact, that I didn't see him again for three-and-a-half years by which time he seemed to be sore again. At one point, veterinary advice had been to remove his anal glands because they were often considered a source of irritation for him, but with regular acupuncture the operation was avoided. Candy could tell the difference and knew it was his back that was bothering him.

It was lovely to see them both again and gratifying that he had done so well. He had a huge reaction to needling his lumbar spine again and snarled and snapped, but after another course of acupuncture (along with treatment for his teeth and anal glands) he was back to running up and down the stairs again. Candy said he was "frisky like a pup" and was delighted at how well he was despite being twelve years old.

The effect of acupuncture can never be predicted. Some animals and people are very sensitive to the needles while others are not. Buddy had a good life until 2014. At fifteen, he had major intestinal problems and nothing could be done.

Most dogs I treat are neutered, but Buddy remains the only one who has been neutered because of his positive response to acupuncture! There are always surprises.

I was thinking of Buddy recently, surprised that five years had passed since he died. I needed Candy's approval about writing his story and wanted to contact her. The first mobile number I tried took me to a recorded message that wasn't Candy, and I almost gave up. But then I found a second file for Buddy and another number. Candy answered. Her voice was as loud and friendly as ever, and she was very pleased to hear from me. Yes, she told me, she would love Buddy's story included in the book 'to immortalise him!'.

Then she said, "I've only got a few weeks left".

I was confused. What was she implying? She sounded so full of life. "I've got ovarian cancer and only a few weeks to live, but I'm fine with it," she continued. I did what I often do – I said how truly sorry I was then put my sadness and shock in a box. She had no regrets – a great life – but if it had been diagnosed sooner things might have been different. She'd been through such a lot. She said I was welcome to visit, and meet her current dog Douglas, and her two cats Watson and Ena.

Time was of the essence. I searched for some photographs of Buddy on my computer and emailed them to her, which delighted her. The one shown of him standing on the consulting room table captures him exactly. And it motivated me to get writing his story. A few days after phoning Candy, I arrived at her door, somewhat apprehensively, wondering how she was keeping because I hadn't heard back from her since emailing her the first draft of Buddy's tale. I was a bit concerned that I might have inadvertently caused her upset with my writing.

When I'd rung to confirm my visit, Candy had told me just to let myself in by the front door. When I stepped into the hallway the house sounded full of people's voices, drowned out by the barking of a dog. Her home-help showed me into the living room, where Candy sat in a hospital chair with her heavily bandaged legs elevated. I immediately noticed the physical change but she welcomed me with her larger-than-life personality. Her tabby cat Ena was draped across the easy chair I was to sit in. Ena was completely unperturbed by Douglas' barking. He was a Lhasa Apso, like Buddy, but he looked quite different. Two of Candy's friends were visiting too, along with their Yorkie, Milly. The warmth in the room was lovely, and it wasn't just due to the heat, and I soaked up the energy and feelings of care and friendship that day.

Candy reminisced about Buddy and events in his life from more than ten years ago. He had just "given up", she told us, before he came for acupuncture, screaming in pain when he was lifted up. She was worried Buddy would have to be cage-rested for most of his life, or be put to sleep. She almost didn't bring him to me, having scoffed when her vet suggested acupuncture. It was only when she found out that her friend's dog, Irish Setter Paddy, was having it and being helped by it that Candy thought she had nothing to lose.

When I mentioned the draft of Buddy's story, she said she hadn't seen it, but promptly found it and read it there and then. What a relief; she laughed a few times and kept saying "That was him! Such a feisty character!". She remembered being astounded by the 'mammoth' change acupuncture had made, how it had "brought him back to life", and how shocked she'd been when he started mounting everything in sight, the embarrassment when he favoured a small child's shoulder. The child thought he was being friendly and cuddly but Candy and his parents looked on in horror. When another friend visited wearing a Clinique perfume, Buddy went into a total frenzy! That's when Candy knew he would have to be neutered.

Amidst all the hilarity caused by Candy's reminiscing, two nurses arrived to attend to her but Candy insisted we stayed put; despite the seriousness of her condition the party atmosphere continued.

"Not everyone gets to cross the door you know", she said. "Only VIPs!"

As I was leaving I said I'd phone to arrange to visit again and she handed me a gift bag containing a 'little something'. It was a beautiful silver trinket box which is in good use to this day, and always reminds me of Candy and Buddy, their special bond and the privilege I had of being part of their lives for a while.

—7—

The lower back and legs

From my years in veterinary practice, I knew how common back pain is in dogs. From my experience with acupuncture in animals, I knew what it could contribute. I was to find just the same with people. There are many leg conditions that are connected to back pain, a common cause of absence from work, and there are multiple factors at play. Most often, the pain is in the lower, lumbosacral area. Nerves can be compressed by degenerating or damaged discs, the cushions between the vertebrae, but pain is often due to muscle tension. Our sedentary lifestyles and hours of sitting at computers or behind the wheel of a car are proven to cause trouble.

Of the many muscles that are involved, there are two large muscle groups that are particular culprits – the quadratus lumborum, which is a large sheet of muscle connecting the pelvis to the lower spine and rib cage, and the gluteal muscles, or glutes, that form the buttock. Using massage to pinpoint the problem areas and soften the muscles, then acupuncture to release yet more tension, often brings great relief. The same is not always true for the very painful complaint of sciatica, but I soon learned how a small but very important muscle near the hip is sometimes responsible.

Scott—sciatica and the piriformis syndrome

There are several causes of sciatica in people, when the large sciatic nerve that runs from the lower spine down the leg becomes irritated with excruciating pain. It can be pinched at different levels, from a bulging (slipped) disc that compresses it where the nerve leaves the spinal canal, or by strained taut muscles along its length. I've never experienced sciatica and hope I never do – I have seen how painful and debilitating it can be.

There is also a specific syndrome caused when the sciatic nerve is entrapped by the piriformis muscle. The nerve usually passes under this small but very powerful muscle which runs from the pelvis to the thigh bone (femur) near the hip. According to a BMAS paper, in around ten percent of people the nerve actually passes through this muscle. If it tightens and squeezes the nerve it can cause the symptoms. Quite appropriately this is called the 'piriformis syndrome'. Releasing the piriformis can relieve the pain and this is where acupuncture comes in.

I had been studying this condition when a twenty-nine-year-old man with a diagnosis of left-side sciatica was referred to me by his GP. Scott was miserable – simply walking caused him great pain. He felt very restricted in what he could do and had been signed off work for a week. He couldn't get comfortable in bed, or lift or play with his young child, and he had stopped going to the gym.

The pain had begun six weeks previously, first with a tight feeling in his left calf which then progressed to pain in his lower back, and travelled down his left leg to his ankle. The leg pain had become more intense than the back pain. Scott knew exactly what had caused it. For eleven years he'd worked as a furniture remover, but six months earlier he'd started spending more time driving and working in the office. The day before the pain started he had lifted a heavy piece of furniture and had felt something in his lower back 'shift'. His doctor had prescribed diclofenac, ibuprofen and co-codamol but they did little to ease the pain. On a visual analogue scale (VAS), he estimated his pain at 83 out of 100.

Using gentle massage I found some tension in Scott's lumbar muscles, but the most painful area was deeper within the left buttock (as shown on the pain map in Fig. 7 *opposite*). The site corresponded to the area of the piriformis muscle – where acupuncture point GB30 lies (Fig. 1). He also had a sore nodule above the left pelvic area. I treated these sites with needles, thinking that a weekly treatment session for four weeks was the best approach.

But he developed 'needle flare' where I'd inserted the needles; his skin became red and he described a "weird sensation of tingling and fluttering" down his left leg, although the treatment wasn't at all painful. He didn't make a second appointment with me at that time because he was unsure of his work commitments, but when I didn't hear from him ten days later I phoned to find out how he was. His wife answered the phone and when I explained who I was there seemed to be a very long pause. Long enough for me to think, "What's happened, has he got worse since the treatment?". Actually, it was completely the opposite. With a voice full of relief she said, "Thank you for giving me back my husband!".

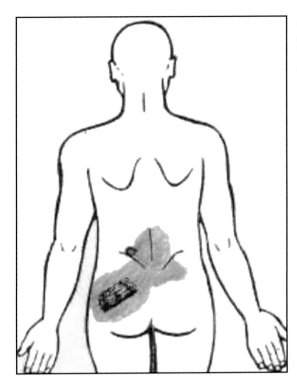

Fig.7: A map of Scott's pain located by massage, showing a round nodule on the left of his lower spine. Hand-drawn by the author.

■ *Major pain*

■ *Minor pain*

Scott had been sore for twenty-four hours following the treatment and had been almost pain-free since, with just a slight twinge in his left leg. He could lift and carry his son again.

"He's a new man!" she told me. He had also stopped taking any medications.

Despite this extremely good response to a single session, I advised her that he would need follow-up, so Scott returned. I was surprised, when massaging him, that I couldn't find any pain – not even in the piriformis area. He still had a non-painful nodule above his iliac crest (the upper part of the pelvis) so this was the only area I needled. I wondered how significant it was, but then Scott remembered he'd had a previous problem with pain and stiffness around the left sacroiliac joint some seven years before, which, we agreed, might have been because of a previous injury.

Three weeks later, Scott came back again. He reported that he'd been pain-free for the first ten days after his last treatment but was still experiencing occasional twinges in his left leg. His VAS estimate was 20 out of 100. This twinge was in a different place, though, going from his hip to the side of his thigh, and was worse when he got into the car. He described it as a tingly pain, like the sensation he'd had when the problem started. He also said he had been busy at work but was coping well. I couldn't identify a painful area, even on the iliac nodule. I decided to include more acupuncture points. When I stimulated GB30 (see Fig. 1), by turning the needle he had an extremely strong twitch response in his gluteal area.

Two weeks later, Scott reported that he was very much better, with only slight intermittent calf pain, and he didn't feel the need for more treatment. Not long after, his colleague came for acupuncture too. He told me that Scott had been fine for months.

Sandra, owner of Brady the Old English Sheepdog

The importance of 'word of mouth' was highlighted yet again when GP David (Chapter 5), after receiving treatment for his neck, recommended acupuncture to his neighbour Sandra. Reminiscing with Sandra, we can't remember who came for treatment first – her, or Brady, her Old English Sheepdog.

What she recalls vividly is the concern she had that Brady was becoming slower and stiffer, and the remarkable difference she noticed after each acupuncture session, when he would bound out of her front door and down the steps, eager for a longer walk. She says she knew then that acupuncture was not a placebo! She could tell from his demeanour when he needed his next session.

Sandra had a good response to acupuncture, too, after being troubled with pain and sciatica related to a spinal disc problem. To avoid a recurrence, she continues to have acupuncture every few weeks, and finds that attending weekly Pilates sessions is helpful.

John the tennis player

John is in his seventies but still plays competitively, occasionally getting twinges in his back. He keeps them at bay by coming for top-up treatments every couple of months. I also insert needles at the acupuncture points for his irritable bowel syndrome (IBS) which stop any flare-ups.

I will say more about the use of acupuncture for conditions other than pain in the next chapter. But of course not every person has such a satisfactory outcome. When someone shows no improvement after four sessions, we usually don't continue.

Alice's hip before resurfacing

Alice was in her late sixties. She had a stiff painful right hip as well as pain in her lower back and groin, necessitating several pain-relieving drugs that she wanted to keep to a minimum. She had severe arthritic changes in her right hip that restricted her range of movement to the point that putting on socks and shoes was a task she dreaded. Alice was waiting for a 'hip resurfacing' operation but it was months away, so she was looking for help to cope with the pain while she waited.

Because she was in so much pain, massage was ruled out. Instead I relied on acupuncture points, away from the hip. After treatment she became more comfortable, and even returned to swimming and started aqua gym twice a week. She was certain that acupuncture had helped lessen her pain and stiffness, allowing her to enjoy exercising in the water once more. She especially felt that cycling in the water helped her perform movements she couldn't do on land. Her quality of life improved greatly before her upcoming surgery.

Ann's knee osteoarthritis and electro-acupuncture in a nonagenarian

At the age of ninety-two, Ann is still my oldest patient. When I first met her, I wondered what acupuncture could do to help at her stage in life. In an ideal world she would have had two knee replacements but, all things considered, her doctors decided against operating, leaving her to manage as best she could. Ann had heard about my acupuncture clinic after her friend attended a talk I gave.

Ann came for her appointments by taxi. She lived alone and was very independent. Apart from the knee pain she was in good health, but I wondered how sensitive she would be to the acupuncture. I winced as she sat down, slowly, and her joints creaked; she quickly assured me that her knees were no more painful than usual. The hospital had taken x-rays of her knees. The left joint was normal, with smooth joint surfaces and space between the bone, but the right one had clear arthritic changes – a narrowed joint space with roughened edges – making the joint less cushioned and less flexible. The x-rays shown overpage are that of a dog, not Ann's, but the changes are exactly the same in humans and dogs!

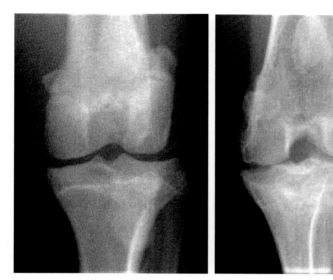

X-ray of a normal knee joint (left) and an osteoarthritic knee joint (right). From the 'Pfizer Atlas of Common Painful Conditions in Dogs and Cats' with permission from Professor Spencer A. Johnston.

After the first session, in which I needled the pain points and points above and below her knee, she hadn't been any sleepier than usual. She felt just fine which I was glad to hear, meaning that she was not overly sensitive to acupuncture. However, there was no difference in her pain. I suggested the use of electro-acupuncture as a stronger form of treatment.

The BMAS electro-acupuncture course I attended in 2007 had covered osteoarthritis of the knee. Much of the research on acupuncture has been done on the treatment of this joint, including the use of electro-acupuncture. A CEFAR ACUS 4™ electric acupuncture stimulator was used on the course. With this system, four pairs of acupuncture needles are connected via crocodile clips to four cables of a power pack. Thankfully, the battery is rechargeable; I once reassured a patient – an electrician – that he wouldn't be connected to the mains supply!

Electro-acupuncture increases the general effect of acupuncture and can be used to treat both acute pain and chronic pain. Sometimes muscle contractions can be seen. The system can be programmed to vary the frequency, pulse and strength of the stimulation, depending on the amplification.

One woman I treated for osteoarthritis in her knees did not like the sensation at all, but Ann loved the feeling, and the treatment took the

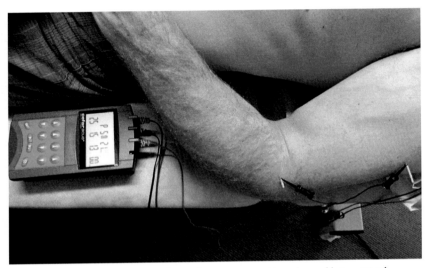

An electro-acupuncture unit. The needles are connected to a chargeable power pack.

edge off her pain for several days and helped her keep on top of it. When she stood up, there was no more creaking. The sense of relief was huge. Determined to keep her independence for as long as possible, she was grateful that electro-acupuncture helped keep her mobile.

George with a sore heel and plantar fasciitis

When it comes to feet there are many conditions for which acupuncture can be used, and some podiatrists use it as part of the treatment they deliver to patients. George had had a sore right heel for over a year, with no idea of the cause. The 'red hot feeling' he described was most intense when he got out of bed and he couldn't put any weight on his heel until the pain had lessened. It didn't disappear, just changed to a bruised feeling, sometimes with pins and needles in his foot. Working part-time as a supply teacher and hospital chaplain, he always had to plan the shortest walking route from A to B, and was frustrated that his weekend rambles were greatly curtailed. His GP suspected plantar fasciitis, and he had been given a steroid injection in his heel and was waiting to see a podiatrist. Unfortunately there had been no improvement after the injection. Ibuprofen was of some help but he didn't want to rely on medication. That was five months before he came to see me. He was totally fed up by that point and his doctor suggested trying acupuncture.

Plantar fasciitis is a common cause of foot pain that can last for months and be very debilitating. It is a chronic form of tendinopathy, characterised by inflammation of the tendons and fascia (layers of thick connective tissue) in the sole or heel of the foot, which can be very painful to touch. There is no recognised best treatment but there are a few options, such as stretching, using sole inserts, steroid injections, massage and acupuncture.

At George's first visit, his foot was extremely painful to touch. There was a sore taut band running across the arch, and his calf and the muscles between the bones in his foot that connect to the toes (metatarsals) were tender on massage. We were both surprised by how widespread his painful areas were (Fig. 8). I used a combination of acupuncture and trigger points on his calf, heel and sole, and recommended gentle stretching exercises for his calf and ankle.

At his second treatment, one week later, George told me that his heel was less sore first thing in the morning, so I extended the treatment area. At the third session, after another ten days, he reported that the foot pain had lessened even more. When I palpated his foot, the area of pain had shifted. Now his Achilles tendon, above the heel, was painful and there was a trigger point at his inside arch.

Another week later, he came for his fourth treatment. By then he was far more comfortable putting his foot down first thing in the

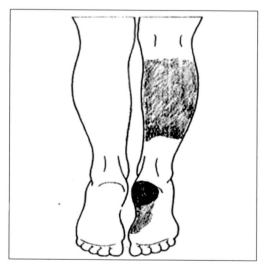

Fig. 8: A map of George's leg pain associated with plantar fasciitis. Hand-drawn by the author.

■ Main area of pain described by George

■ Additional areas of pain found on palpation

morning, and the pins and needles had gone completely. But although his heel was less painful, it still felt bruised. I couldn't find any specific area of pain in his heel but I did at the ball and upper part of his foot. George had seen the podiatrist by then, who recommended calf exercises for tendinitis, and called him back in three months' time.

Around three weeks later George reported that his heel had been feeling so good on normal daily use that he had gone hiking two days before coming to the clinic. There was no pain in his calf muscles this time, but he was sore again, with painful gristly trigger points on the sole of his foot, at the arch. I treated this.

The soreness of his heel eventually went, and George felt that the improvement was due to acupuncture. He never got into the habit of stretching, but did start doing some exercises along with the acupuncture, which were also beneficial. Six months later, he reported that after the last acupuncture session his heel had only been mildly uncomfortable for a few weeks. He had started doing calf exercises regularly, and was wearing a Scholl™ shoe insert. For the previous four months he had had no heel pain at all.

I was taught that trigger points in the calf muscles can often lead to foot pain. While George was one of my earlier cases, it highlighted the importance of examining a wider area than just the obviously sore bit. Liz, one of the GPs at the clinic, knows this is very important when examining a patient, but says she only fully appreciated the fact through her acupuncture training. She thinks more emphasis should be made on seeking the source of muscular pain in medical-school courses.

A vet friend asked me if I thought the same applies when it comes to animals. In my opinion, there is a key difference in as much that an animal cannot describe its pain, so vets rely much more on making a very comprehensive physical examination.

It appeared that George's tight calf muscles had been pulling on the plantar fascia in his foot, but I have never had two cases the same. In Chapter 12, I describe another case of foot pain which was more unusual, and this person came to me because of their dog!

As plantar fasciitis is a frequent cause of foot pain in the patients I see, I completed a study of its treatment and also made a comparison of acupuncture protocols. Along with a review of the use of acupuncture in veterinary medicine, which I sent to all the UK and Dublin veterinary schools in an attempt to encourage its use, I received a postgraduate

Certificate in Western Medical Acupuncture from the University of Hertfordshire. That was back in 2012. I progressed using acupuncture and became more convinced of its value in both veterinary and medical fields, yet there was still so much doubt among the professional bodies. In 2010 I wrote a letter to the *Veterinary Record* to encourage the use of acupuncture. This resulted in two very scathing replies, which were also published. In contrast, I received two emails, both of which were very supportive. One was from a female vet who had suffered chronic pain after a riding accident; acupuncture had been an invaluable part of her recovery. For every negative response or two, there is always a positive story or event in contradiction, which has kept me on the acupuncture path. One of these is Bob's story.

Bob's sore elbow

As plantar fasciitis is a tendinitis, it has a lot of similarities to tennis elbow and golfer's elbow. Neither condition is necessarily linked to sport! Bob is a hill-walking (but non-tennis playing) friend. He had been plagued by a sore elbow, typical of tennis elbow, for many months.

Acupuncture worked wonders for him. The one and only acupuncture session we managed to fit in to his busy schedule elicited a huge twitch in the muscle just below his elbow; the pain subsequently went away and never came back. If only every case were as straightforward as this one!

— 8 —

You cannot be serious!

At the BMAS conference at a hotel in Newcastle, a doctor asked me about treating animals with acupuncture and the positive outcomes that were reported by their owners.

"There must be a placebo effect on the owner, then," he said.

I was taken aback as I tried to take his comments on board. I thought about the placebo effect. Originating from Latin meaning 'I shall please', placebo now refers to a positive effect obtained from an inert substance due to the mind believing that the substance will help. We accept that there is an element of the placebo effect in humans – not just for acupuncture but many other treatments – because our mind is a powerful tool. I was at a veterinary talk once, where someone commented that the placebo effect may account for up to sixty per cent of the effect painkillers have in humans.

It has been shown that the outcome is better with acupuncture if the acupuncturist discusses, listens and takes time with the patient, compared with an acupuncturist entering a room, inserting the needles and leaving without saying a word. This suggests that the motions of acupuncture alone are less effective; and this is why sugar-pill placebos instead of an active medicine sometimes make a person feel better. But is it the same with animals?

I felt instantly defensive about the doctor's words, with their implication that we were hoodwinking the animals' owners. It's safe to assume that, unlike a human patient, an animal neither knows why it is at the vets, nor has any expectations about the treatment. Yet the treatment might stop a limp. It seems like a genuine effect. It is true that owners can be overly optimistic during the first couple of sessions, but if there is no improvement in their pet after around four sessions, we do not continue.

Owners have to commit to making appointments and consider the costs, so a good result is important, which must be measurable. There are systems based on an animal's behaviour and level of mobility that give a pain score in order to evaluate the effectiveness of treatments and overall quality of life. They are more often used for hospitalised animals or research purposes. In the clinic setting it is just as useful to note the observations and changes of certain behaviours and motion.

Dogs and cats have to have some degree of trust to allow acupuncture to be carried out, even though most needle points are not painful. But as with people there can be an 'ouch' response – what the Chinese call an *Ah Qi* or *De Qi* response. The animal may try to get away momentarily, or at worst turn to bite. Again, the animal has no expectation that the treatment will work.

What is known is that acupuncture causes the body to release feel-good substances like serotonin, oxytocin and endorphins, so perhaps some animals associate the visit simply with feeling good. And getting a treat from the vet also helps! Others never lose their apprehension and won't even take a treat. It's lovely to see them become less anxious and confident enough to accept one!

The doctor's question made me think of a particular case when, in my opinion, the power of acupuncture could not be disputed.

All singing and dancing (ASAD) points

In 2007 I was at another medical acupuncture training day, this time about palliative care, where we learnt about the 'All Singing and Dancing' or ASAD points that could be used for controlling symptoms. The 'A' stands for anxiety, 'S' for sickness, the second 'A' for analgesia (pain control) and 'D' is for dyspnoea (breathing problems). These are two points high up on the upper section of the breastbone, near the neck, an area known as the manubrium, which the lecturer often used in combination with needles placed at the web of the thumbs (point LI4) and near the big toes (point LR3).

The hospital auditorium was packed for the lecture, but with a settled air. The lecturer explained how, for some patients, acupuncture is very effective for alleviating symptoms of some conditions when all pharmaceutical options have been exhausted or stopped because of side-effects. We heard about the theories, but it was listening to the patients talking that had the most impact on me. Gordon's case was the most vivid. We had just finished lunch, and it would have been easy to nod off had the topic not been so riveting. The lights went up and the doctor moved from behind the lectern to the bench at centre stage while we waited for the patient to enter.

We were told that Gordon (not his real name) had had extensive and prolonged treatment for throat cancer – surgery followed by chemotherapy and radiotherapy. He now suffered from chronic pain because of tissue damage. Acupuncture didn't take his pain away completely but regular top-up treatments had a cumulative effect and his pain lessened.

The doctor told us what was going to happen. Gordon would sit on the bench and she would insert needles along the back of his shoulders and neck. She told us that Gordon might lose consciousness, at which point the needles would be quickly removed. He would then sleep for several minutes. That was his treatment.

From my seat towards the back of the auditorium, I realised I was sitting with my arms crossed defensively as I tried to reconcile my thoughts. Here was one of the most experienced doctors in the field telling me something I struggled to believe. Gordon duly entered the room and began to tell his story, speaking through a voice box because of the damage to his larynx. Every type of painkiller had been tried, but they hadn't made much difference. His life hadn't been worth living, and he'd planned to jump from the window of his flat in a high-rise block. He told us he was only alive still because acupuncture had eased his pain and made his life bearable.

It happened exactly as the doctor described. Gordon sat in the middle of the bench with the doctor behind him and an assistant either side of the bench. As Gordon was passing out, the needles were quickly removed and the assistants safely guided him into a lying position. The auditorium was hushed, as was my naysayer voice. I was completely hooked, and felt a surge of commitment to the welfare of patients, whether animal or human, flow through my whole body.

There was no way I could let acupuncture be swept aside by cynical vets and doctors claiming there was no evidence for its powerful effect, and there was no way I would let myself get so wrapped up with conventional veterinary work to have no time for it. From that moment on I was determined to continue learning and exploring what acupuncture could do and how I could best use it for the patients that crossed my path.

I often felt I was being taught by my patients. The following animal cases proved to me that acupuncture helps in conditions other than pain, when all the conventional treatments had failed, and I least expected it to work.

The mystery of Cloud's skin

Cloud the cat (also known as Bertie) looked like the alien E.T. in the movie! Vet Rachel had tried everything to treat Cloud's itchy skin condition. Biopsy had given a likely diagnosis of an eosinophilic dermatitis – an immune reaction with no cure, requiring symptomatic control with steroids. It wasn't a long-term solution because of the potential side effects, but it did help to suppress the reaction, so that Cloud itched less and licked less, allowing the scabby lumps to reduce a bit.

"What can acupuncture do?" Rachel asked me.

The fact that Cloud's skin problem had been waxing and waning for years alerted my internal naysayer once more, but I'd been to that remarkable lecture and had seen what acupuncture had done for Gordon.

Cloud's owner Carol was a dietitian in a diabetes clinic and thought, when acupuncture was suggested by Rachel for Cloud's skin, that she was either taking the mickey, or things had got so desperate it was a joke. When Rachel explained that it was a *serious* option, Carol decided to go ahead despite her scepticism. She wondered how on earth Cloud was going to tolerate needles.

When I saw Cloud for myself, the naysayer inside me had a field day. There he was, with his bald face, over-sized ears and a long scraggy neck all covered in lumps; and on closer inspection, his body was also covered in lumps. The condition was certainly chronic.

Cloud was only three years old when he started to lose hair around his neck and began a long association with steroid, hormone and antibiotic treatments. Other things troubled him too. His anal (scent) glands didn't empty themselves; instead they filled up and irritated him, and he hated having them expressed by squeezing.

When his stomach went bald it was found he had the fungal infection ringworm, which also needed treatment. Once he came home with a damaged tail that required surgery. And on top of all this, it was anticipated that his knees were going to cause a problem with arthritis at some point.

The skin problem persisted. Raised lumps appeared on his legs and the skin was particularly red and irritated, so a sample of a lump was taken. The pathology results suggested an insect bite, but this happened mid-winter making that an unlikely diagnosis.

By the time I saw Cloud he was thirteen, and also had bowel and liver issues. He wasn't a good candidate for general anaesthesia or surgical investigation. The number of lumps on his face and body had increased in both size and number. More samples were taken for a more accurate diagnosis that might lead to better treatment. The results were inconclusive, indicating a type of eosinophilic granuloma complex, an inflammatory condition.

The Royal (Dick) School of Veterinary Studies at Edinburgh University (known widely as the Dick Vet) were contacted for advice. Chemotherapy could sometimes help but was not indicated in Cloud's case. I knew that acupuncture could affect the immune system, so it was worth a try.

I examined Cloud's threadbare bald skin which was thickened and rough to the touch with small lumps all over. It was difficult to imagine what he should look like – he was meant to be grey. The worst part was his bleeding scabby right ear.

Carol and I remember that Cloud was very relaxed and didn't mind acupuncture at all. He tolerated all the points I chose to stimulate his immune system with no problem. To our amazement, even after only two sessions, the changes started to occur.

His ear dried up and the scabbiness reduced. Carol also noticed a change in his behaviour; he seemed to have more energy and was more sociable. Over time, the fur around his eyes grew back and he started getting furrier elsewhere. All but a single lump shrank and eventually disappeared. His steroid tablets were reduced then stopped altogether. It got to a stage where only a monthly acupuncture top-up was needed. That remaining lump, on his right ear, was more like fatty tissue than an inflammatory response and he was completely unaware of it so didn't scratch.

Carol described the results as 'spectacular'. We wondered what might have happened with Cloud's woes if we had tried acupuncture much earlier. I regret that I don't have 'before' and (what would have been impressive) 'after' photographs to include in this book; I didn't bother recording the state he was in because I hadn't expected any improvements.

Cloud taught both Rachel and me that even in the face of adversity, acupuncture should be tried. The successful outcome led us to try another challenging case.

Tiny Kizi's liver

I knew all about Yorkshire terrier Kizi. She was notorious in the practice for being particularly difficult to handle, and I couldn't believe it when Rachel suggested acupuncture. Kizi had a liver condition and every so often she went off her food, and became lethargic and miserable. Blood results showed that her liver enzymes were elevated, indicating a recurrent hepatitis. She was regularly hospitalised for a few days at a time to get supportive treatment, but giving her intravenous fluids was difficult because a catheter needed to be inserted into a vein, which is tricky in a small leg attached to a squirming body. Despite weighing only three kilograms, Kizi didn't want to be handled. She would recover and be fine for a few months until the next bout of illness. We always knew when she was ready to go home because she became so 'vocal'.

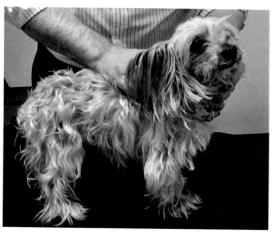

A very small Kizi, weighing just 3 kilograms.

Thus Kizi was far from being an ideal acupuncture patient. Some of the recommended points for stimulating liver function are on the abdomen, near to the umbilicus (equivalent to our tummy button). Spaniel Griff had been the only animal with liver problems I had experience of treating, and because he had done so well it was only fair to try with Kizi. Her owners Mark and Kay were hopeful it would work.

The day arrived and Kizi seemed even smaller – so very dainty, with a long unkempt coat. She hated being groomed but that seemed to be the least of her problems. When she came into the room she was already protesting loudly, and before I even started the treatment Kay left the room because she was so anxious! Mark stayed with me as Kizi continued to react to simply being held. My heart sank, but Mark was confident he could hold her. Kizi was going through one of her better spells, so the question was could we use acupuncture preventitively, to stop her liver enzymes from elevating by healing or stimulating liver function in some way?

Mark cuddled her close as I tried just a few acupuncture points on her back to see how she tolerated it. It went remarkably well. At the next session I wanted to add some abdominal points but even with Mark cuddling her she gave a high-pitched scream – totally unexpected from such a tiny dog. She certainly had spirit, but hearing that made me feel awful, and the people outside in the waiting room must have wondered what was going on. I had to aim as close to the tummy points as I could but of course my target was moving and I couldn't be as precise as I would have liked. But as Mark reminisced some years later, "Kizi could scream like a small child before she had any needles!".

I never felt comfortable treating Kizi and frankly would have preferred not to, but Mark always reassured me that her anxiety was short-lived, and she recovered straight after the session. Carrying out acupuncture is usually calming and pleasant but with Kizi it felt anything but. She didn't understand that it was for her benefit (there was definitely no placebo effect with her). Vet Rachel was keen to continue – it was working and I was to keep going.

However, Kizi never got used to acupuncture! We increased the gap between her treatments as quickly as possible, first to every six weeks, then to every eight, and Mark and Kay saved heaps on hospitalisation expenses! Kay was so impressed that she contacted a newspaper, although the reporters didn't follow the story up. Over the following two years Kizi only came into the hospital once, when she and the two other family dogs feasted on a rotting sea-bird carcass on the beach and ended up with a nasty bout of toxic gastroenteritis causing vomiting and diarrhoea.

The cause of Kizi's liver problem was never discovered – that would have involved yet further interventions and biopsies– but acupuncture kept her going, giving her a far better quality of life. Amazingly, she reached the age of sixteen.

And Sweep's liver ...

My vet colleague Rachel later brought her own dog Sweep to me, who also had a liver condition. This time, it was a chronic active hepatitis. Sweep was a Cockapoo (a Spaniel crossed with a Poodle) who often lost her appetite and even refused a treat when she arrived for treatment. But immediately after acupuncture, she guzzled down her treats and was able to jump on the bed again!

Keeping on top of Finn's pancreatitis

Finn's owner Lorraine already had experience of acupuncture. Her other dog, a Giant Schnauzer called Fairin, had been coming for a long time for back treatment, and he was a star patient. He got so used to coming that he would amble into the consulting room and lie down on his side without being asked, legs outstretched and hardly moved for the duration of his appointment. It was a bit unhelpful, however, when he was in for a routine check-up or vaccination and confused the vet by taking up his usual position

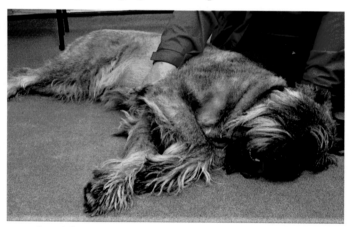

Giant Schnauzer Fairin always took up this position when he came to the vets – expecting to get acupuncture!

When Lorraine's Miniature Schnauzer, Finn, was recovering from a bout of pancreatitis, she asked if acupuncture would help. Pancreatitis is a very painful and serious illness involving inflammation of the pancreas and the release of excess digestive enzymes. There's always a worry that it will return because sometimes we have no idea what set it off in the first place.

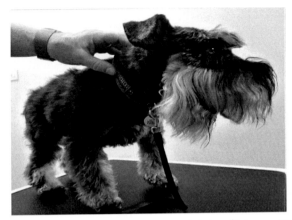

Miniature Schnauzer Finn – acupuncture attempts to keep his pancreatitis at bay.

It was likely that Finn was going to be on lifetime medication, with no guarantee that the condition wouldn't return, but we introduced acupuncture alongside this. More than four years have now passed since Finn's last serious bout and he only comes for acupuncture once every three months. Our fingers stay crossed.

Darcy and Millie at the end of life

Rachel was apologetic because of the condition of one of her patients when she explained to me why she wanted to try acupuncture. It was a last resort for Lakeland Terrier Darcy. Her owner Brenda's situation was compounded by the fact she had another chronically ill dog at home, Millie, who was the same breed. It was sad to have two dogs nearing the end of life at the same time, but Brenda was stoic and made the most of the situation. Both dogs were getting the best of care at the Inglis vet practice, where Rachel now worked, and a specialist veterinary referral centre, but Rachel wanted to try out all possible treatment options.

Some cases are tricky because they make you question the concept of 'quality of life' and how we measure it and the ethics of prolonging life when the quality is poor. This is sure to become an even bigger issue as medical technology and treatments advance. I read Darcy's history and prepared to meet her. Hers was a complex case, with a history of pancreatitis and advanced kidney failure. Her owner Brenda worked as a home-carer and hated injections and needles, but she duly put her reservations aside to keep up with Darcy's medications. Because of the extreme circumstances Brenda had been taught not just how to syringe fluids by mouth, but also to inject them under the skin so Darcy could be cared for at home. Yet, despite all this special care, Darcy was reluctant to eat or drink and was so thin and lethargic when I saw her that I held out little hope. I began Darcy's acupuncture treatment, and she became brighter overall. Still some ups and downs, but the most convincing improvement was that she put on two kilograms in weight over two months. Her specialist vet was amazed!

For a while both of Brenda's dogs came together for acupuncture – Darcy received eight months and Millie four months of acupuncture. Both lived beyond our veterinary expectations. Brenda enjoyed that extra time with her dogs, and they enjoyed a better quality of life.

Neurological problems for Sean, Riva, Barney and Skye

Neurological cases involving nerve damage or degeneration can be very difficult to treat; in theory, for acupuncture to work best an intact nervous system is needed. Sean the Rottweiler was one of my early cases using acupuncture post-operatively. At ten years of age he'd been partially paralysed by a bulging cervical disc and had specialist surgery to remove some bone and decompress the spinal cord. At one time, operating on a ten-year old dog would not be recommended, but people and pets all live longer now with a better quality of life, and Sean was in great shape. Hydrotherapy would have been good for his rehabilitation after surgery, but he wasn't a swimmer so it was ruled out. Acupuncture it was, then.

Sean was very uncoordinated because he had ataxia. He walked as if he were drunk and dribbled urine when I saw him six weeks after his surgery. Otherwise his recovery was going according to plan and his owner Jean was keen to help him as much as possible. Luckily Sean was sensitive to acupuncture, giving a lively twitch response to needles along his back, but remaining unfazed. After eleven treatments over a six-month period, he could cock his leg again and walk straighter and more upright. His hind legs only swayed a little when he turned a corner. By this time Jean was no longer regarding him as a 'patient', having seen an improvement immediately after each session. Obviously the surgery had been a great success but acupuncture was a good adjunct to his recovery, and may well have speeded it up.

It can be very serious when weakness of a hind limb is caused by nerve degeneration – usually nothing can be done. So when I was faced with treating Miniature Schnauzer, Riva, I was unsure what the effect of acupuncture would be because of her history.

Riva was approaching thirteen years of age when she had fallen on the stairs, leaving her hind legs a bit unsteady. When examined, her reflexes were poor. When her back paws were placed in a 'knuckled' position, she didn't instantly correct their position, which was a sure sign that the messages from her brain were not reaching her paws. Just in case a disc in her spine was pressing on a nerve, rest and meloxicam were advised even though she did not seem to be in pain.

For a year, Riva had occasional bouts of unsteadiness but these had worsened. Her walking was slow, her back was hunched, she had difficulty squatting for the toilet and was generally unhappy. When Riva had been hospitalised, pain was located in her thoracolumbar spine (Fig. 3), so x-rays were taken which revealed significant spondylosis at the junction of the spine with the pelvis (the lumbosacral or LS area). It was worse at the level of the last ribs.

Her owner Linda was thinking there was no hope of improvement for Riva, but her friend had suggested she try acupuncture. Riva's vet, Neil, a partner in the practice, was still unconvinced. And he was not the only one. Even I had little hope that acupuncture would do anything for nerve damage. Linda later told me I had been very explicit with her.

"Acupuncture is well worth trying," I had said. "But I think only two sessions because it may not do anything," However, after the very first session Linda proudly described Riva bouncing around the garden like a new spring lamb! Riva walked more or less in a straight line and she never looked back! Riva reached the amazing age of seventeen. After three years of acupuncture it was heart failure – not her mobility– that was her downfall.

When I saw how chocolate Labrador Barney was walking, I was reminded of Riva. He was also ataxic, but not as badly. Jim and Anne, his owners, had recently noticed that he dragged his hind legs on occasion and they heard his paws scuffing along the floor. Barney was approaching ten years. He had been x-rayed at his practice and Anne and Colin didn't want him to undergo any further investigations – because, despite his faulty hind legs, he was happy!

The x-rays showed spondylosis of some of his thoracic vertebrae with bony changes in the lumbosacral (LS) area. In contrast, his lumbar vertebrae were well spaced out with no signs of spondylosis. The fuzzy outline where the spine meets the pelvis on Barney's x-ray shows typical arthritic changes that are commonly seen in older dogs (and similar to previous case Riva), which may contribute to stiffness and discomfort in the area.

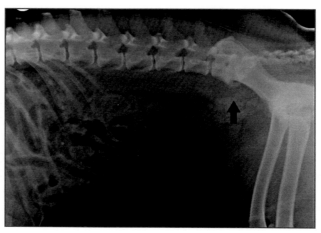

*An x-ray of Barney's lumbosacral changes. Courtesy of
Kingdom Veterinary Clinic*

The x-ray didn't explain Barney's neurological changes but it did rule out an obvious disc problem – or a tumour or a change in bone density. Again I still questioned what acupuncture could do for him.

As it turns out, it was quite a lot! Barney showed no signs of pain when I felt the joints of his hind limbs, but the muscles along his back were tight. He made himself at home on the floor and turned out to be another ideal candidate. With twitches along his spine (and one or two bent needles due to the muscle release), Barney showed an immediate response. After his first two sessions he was jumping up the three steps of the back door of the house, which Anne and Jim thought he would never be able to do again, and he was scuffing his feet less and was generally much happier in himself.

Barney continues with acupuncture every two months and has also lost around four kilograms in weight, which is a big help (Jim and Anne discovered that he loves carrots as much as biscuits!). He rarely

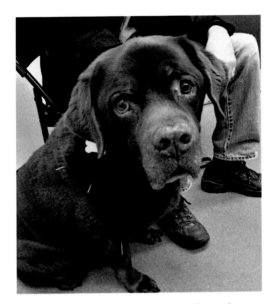

Barney at ease with acupuncture needles in place.

scuffs his feet now and hasn't needed regular anti-inflammatory medication for two years. Twelve years old and still going strong – yet another reminder that for some cases presenting with ataxia for which pharmaceuticals do not help, acupuncture might.

Sam was a black Labrador who had visited over the years for acupuncture to help with his arthritic joints. On those visits, I would hear about Skye, Susan the owner's other dog, a chocolate Labrador, who was having chemotherapy. Skye had successful cancer treatment from vet Simon who worked alongside the Dick vet school. Skye's problems were completely different from Sam's. Acupuncture had helped Sam with his pain and stiffness, but Skye didn't seem to be in any pain, however her right hind leg was getting weaker; the muscles in her right thigh were losing their tone because the nerve supply was deteriorating for some unknown reason. Susan wasn't keen to pursue further investigation, as Skye was essentially happy and enjoying her life.

I thought of previous difficulties I'd had with a neurological case. That was Eddie, a Collie-cross belonging to vet Emma. When his hind limbs deteriorated similarly, we tried electro-acupuncture on him. Unfortunately he worsened, albeit temporarily, possibly due to exacerbated muscle fatigue, and he became wobblier and more uncoordinated. It was a sobering thought. So with Skye I decided not to use electro-acupuncture. She was one of those cases where I didn't expect much more, yet standard acupuncture stopped the deterioration and she was able to hold her own. Later hydrotherapy was added to her treatment regimen, which helped maintain the strength of her hind legs, clearly measurable by how well she coped with getting into a car.

Susan felt that Skye lived far longer than expected, until the inevitable day when she couldn't stand up anymore. Susan is now contemplating whether the time may be right to get another dog, although now she has her own diagnosis to contend with. There is often a link between treating a pet and then their owner, and vice versa, which is how it went with Susan and her dogs.

Susan has pulmonary fibrosis, where for some reason her lungs have lost their elasticity. There is no drug treatment. So far, she is the only patient with this condition I have attempted to treat. Monthly acupuncture alongside her physiotherapy helps, she tells me, and said of her latest treatment:

"I can't believe the difference I felt after my acupuncture this time. It was the best yet! I felt as if I was raring to go and went to my physio the next day with a skip in my step".

At the time of writing her lung capacity is stable.

— 9 —

Strong responders and
laser acupuncture

Some animals and people have instant reactions to acupuncture. The most memorable from my point of view is undoubtedly the human patient in the auditorium I saw passing out when the needles were inserted across his shoulders (in Chapter 8). Then there was Mandy, the vet, and her sweaty palm. And two canine cases also left their mark (on my memory, luckily not on my skin)!

Sisko and a close call for my fingers!

I had never met a Belgian Shepherd before, a smaller shaggier version of a German Shepherd, but Yvonne had several and loved them above all other dogs. She was a successful breeder who had won plenty of prizes at shows. At that time she had seven of them at home. I was catching up with Yvonne and remembering Sisko. She said she would never forget the look on my face at Sisko's huge reaction during his acupuncture treatment, when he came close to biting me. That was twelve years ago. For the first eight years of his life, apart from regular vaccination, including the rabies one so he could qualify for a pet passport and travel to shows abroad, Sisko was hardly ever at the vets. He had been Show Champion and along with his placid nature was one of Yvonne's favourites.

Then, when he turned eight, Yvonne noticed something was wrong. Sisko was sitting down in the show ring at inopportune moments and didn't want to walk far. For a couple of days after, he was a bit unsteady on his hind legs so Yvonne brought him to the practice for examination. I found some painful areas on his spine and thought this was where the problem lay; saying that, he also had a reduced appetite and weight loss that indicated something else was going on. Nothing showed up on the tests, though. He just wasn't himself and Yvonne was very worried. Because her husband Alan had benefited from acupuncture after a back injury, Yvonne was happy to give it a go with Sisko.

When I first saw Sisko there had been some improvement over the previous month, with rest, time and medication. Her vet, the boss at the practice, was now recommending acupuncture and hydrotherapy. Sisko was better at placing his feet but Yvonne still had to help him stand by lifting his hind end. When he tried to run, he bunny-hopped and held his tail rigid, and it was sometimes difficult for him to balance while cocking his leg. He was also eating better and had just started climbing the steps in the garden again. But he still wasn't shaking or scratching himself as he usually did.

My plan was to treat his spine and see if this was at the root of his problems. Yvonne only wanted him to be x-rayed if it were absolutely necessary. If the cause was muscular, nothing would show up on x-ray anyway. I was aware Sisko was improving, albeit slowly.

I didn't want to stimulate any painful response as I examined him so I gently felt along his spine. All I could feel was a small gristly area in the left thoracolumbar area (at the end of the rib cage; see Fig. 3). As Sisko calmly stood on the floor with Yvonne at his head end, I began inserting needles along both sides of his back, near his tail, planning to work upwards to what might be the problem area. Sisko was totally unfazed, and I hadn't delivered my usual warning about the bite response. Luckily, as I worked closer, I just remembered to tell Yvonne that sometimes reactions can be powerful if a needle elicits a strong 'ouch' response, and that even the nicest dog can bite. I am forever grateful that she tightened her hold on either side of his neck just as I inserted a needle on his right side, opposite the gristly area. Although I did this only very superficially, Sisko had one of the strongest reactions I've ever seen. His head swept round and he tried to lunge towards me while snapping. He was so fast! He hadn't reacted at all to the previous needles but obviously I had found a trigger point, and he wanted to tell me about it!

Sisko settled down again quickly and I took the needle out, but it took Yvonne and me a lot longer to get over our fright! It still amazes me that even with such a strong reaction, the pain is very fleeting and the 'ouch' moment seems to go instantly. With Sisko, the fact that, along with his surprising response, two of the needles on his right side were bent meant that some very taut muscles were lurking beneath. When very tight muscle fibres contract then suddenly release, they can move in different directions, which the thin needles can't withstand. I was sure the hypersensitivity boded well for Sisko, but my plan was to arrange more blood tests and x-rays of his spine and hips if he didn't get better or there was any deterioration.

As it turns out, Yvonne reported lots of changes for the better when they came back two weeks later. The bunny-hopping was still there, but Sisko was managing to shake himself, cock his leg and move his tail more. I needled him again, and he reacted in the same area, this time with a little yelp and only one needle was bent. By his third session over three weeks, as well as hydrotherapy, Sisko was returning to his confident self, far more active and even managing to walk up steep banks. Two weeks later, at his fourth session, Yvonne was amazed how well he had been; he was doing things he hadn't done for a very long time and his anti-inflammatory medication had been reduced by half. At the next visit, Yvonne described him as a new dog. He was able to stop his medication and we planned to follow up with maintenance sessions, two months apart. Taut muscles can tighten up again but a combination of acupuncture and hydrotherapy would hopefully keep them free. Sisko was back to his former glory, and Yvonne was delighted when he got back in the show-ring and began winning prizes as a veteran!

She reduced his food intake to help him lose weight, while the hydrotherapy helped him burn off calories and strengthen the muscles in his hind limbs. As he got stronger, he spent longer in the pool and was able to put in more effort. For the next two years, he kept up with the hydrotherapy and acupuncture top-up every two or three months, not coming to the vets for anything else other than his vaccinations.

Sadly, he only reached the age of ten. A devastated Yvonne found him collapsed in the garden one morning, and she and Alan were unable to revive him. There had been no warning – he'd seemed perfectly well. Without an autopsy, there was no telling what the cause was – perhaps he had an undetected heart problem. The only comfort is that Sisko had not suffered from an illness and Yvonne and Alan were spared the decision of having him put to sleep.

Nell's transformation!

Nell the black Lab came confidently down the sloping passageway, but her head was nodding – a sure sign of significant forelimb lameness. This was her first visit for acupuncture and my first meeting with her and her owner Lorna. X-rays had shown mild to moderate arthritic change in both elbow joints over a year before, but the damage wasn't considered enough to explain her persistent left-side limp.

A sample of joint fluid hadn't revealed any infection but it was typical of degenerative osteoarthritis. The referring vet thought it was worth seeing what acupuncture could do to help as there had been little change with medication, and sorting out her medication was difficult because anti-inflammatory treatments made her vomit and gave her diarrhoea. Lorna followed the vet's advice, which helped Nell to begin with. Now she had lost some weight, her exercise had been reduced and she was on a joint supplement and Symmetrel™ (amantadine) for the pain of progressive osteoarthritis). Latterly she seemed unhappy and her limp was worse. She was stiffest in the mornings and reluctant to get out of bed. Sometimes she just couldn't be bothered and had even lost interest in going up to the field where Lorna kept her horses. Later, Lorna told me how sceptical she had been about acupuncture and that she had put it off for some time. Nell's reaction to it was a surprise to us both – in bad and good ways!

After getting a biscuit, Nell got up onto the low-level elevating table and was raised up to a comfortable height for Lorna and me to start work. She lay on her side and then fully on her back with her paws in the air, relaxed, trusting and submissive. I had never seen a dog do this before on a first visit. Lorna laughed and said, "You can do anything with her!".

Over the years, having seen a huge variety of dogs, and if I had to say which type of dog was best suited for acupuncture I would say Labradors – black ones! Being a black Labrador, I had every confidence that Nell would be fine with the process, and at first that's how it seemed to be. As she lay there, I used some initial introductory points along her back to test her reaction and was able to treat around and inside her left elbow. There were twitches from the needles at her elbow and the front of her shoulder, and more twitching behind her shoulder. But when I hit a point in the triceps muscle, she let out a deep-throated growl, so I removed the needle instantly. It gave Lorna and I quite a fright, but Lorna was truly shocked because she had never heard Nell growl like that. Nell seemed to forget about it quickly and became quite sleepy. She yawned as she got off the table. I felt, with a reaction like that, that if acupuncture was going to help it was going to have to work quickly. It must have felt like an electric shock to Nell, but it clearly pinpointed that the pain in her shoulder was in a muscle rather than a joint.

I had told Lorna that if the needle hits a sore spot then anything can happen, and it seemed that Nell was very sensitive. When we made the next appointment, I doubted Lorna would return. A week later, however, Nell and Lorna were back! Nell was striding down the passageway as confidently as ever, as if nothing had happened, and her gait was smooth – no limp! Lorna was delighted and so was I!

For two days after the acupuncture, Lorna told me, Nell still had her usual limp, but then it went away. She said Nell was bouncier and seemed happier. At this session, I treated the same area near the triceps shoulder point, which was fine, but she growled about a knee point that I used to help her front leg.

As the acupuncture had such a marked effect, I made the third appointment for two weeks later rather than one. The positive effect lasted and by the time of that third treatment, Nell was bounding up to the horse field again, way ahead of Lorna instead of lagging behind. After just two sessions of acupuncture Nell had been transformed. She didn't just stop limping – her whole demeanour had changed and her vitality was back.

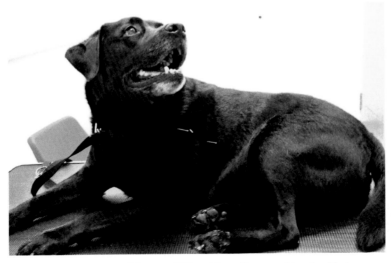

A very trusting and forgiving Nell – with needles around her shoulder!

She came for a third time. I was aware how sensitive she was and that growling was very unusual for Nell, but she had an even bigger reaction during this visit. I started with superficial needles away from her left foreleg and came along her back. She gave a small growl at the knee point, but when I reached a point at her left shoulder, a spot in the middle of the triceps muscle between her shoulder and elbow, she growled and snapped. It was the closest I have ever come to being bitten during an acupuncture session. I was shocked but my reflexes were quick enough to get me out of the way, but I had felt her teeth against my skin. Nell had given me a warning, and she looked frightened.

Lorna was utterly horrified. She had never seen Nell react like that – ever. The treatment came to an abrupt end, but I certainly wasn't going to do any more that day. I had nearly finished anyway, so she didn't miss out on much. I felt so sorry that I had caused her so much pain, even briefly. Nell was such a trusting soul and didn't understand what we were trying to do.

We increased the interval between her visits to two months and used a muzzle on a couple of occasions, but she never had such a strong response again. She continued to be very sensitive and often had twitch responses at her back and left shoulder, with just the occasional growl. She growled one time because I had to remove a tick from her head at the same time!

Over the next three years, Nell came for top-ups every six to eight weeks, not the usual four weeks, and for all that time she stayed very well other than a mild bout of suspected pancreatitis. She slowed down, though, and generally became stiffer over time but she coped well, until one day she became lame on her left hind leg.

Lorna had noticed some changes over the previous month and that Nell's left hind leg was bothering her. Sometimes she needed help to get up on her hind legs, and she was lethargic. She had also lost weight, which rang alarm bells. Vet Simon and I both suspected an arthritic flare-up in the left knee, where some years ago she had had a TPLO operation (tibial plateau levelling osteotomy) to repair the cruciate ligament and stabilise the joint. We decided to investigate further, so Nell was x-rayed under anaesthetic. The only change in her blood results was a mild increase in liver enzymes, so we knew that Nell's metabolism was fine. However, the x-ray revealed an unusually large aggressive bone tumour on the left side of her pelvis. Sadly, Lorna had to make the decision to let her go. Nell was euthanised peacefully, surrounded by her family at home.

Both Nell and Sisko had strong reactions when their taut muscles were released instantly by needling, and subsequently became more tolerant of the treatment. However, some animals and people are so sensitive to needling, that for them laser treatment is the best option.

Laser treatment

I recently found out that the word 'laser' is an acronym. It stands for 'light amplification by the stimulated emission of radiation'. Essentially lasers use light energy. There are many different types used in human and veterinary medicine to stimulate the healing process and reduce pain and inflammation. Its action differs from acupuncture, although both work at a cellular level.

In 2012, at another BMAS conference, a paediatrician introduced us to the use of lasers. What sticks in my mind the most was his description of treating children with eczema that was so severe that they had to be hospitalised. The painless treatment with a laser helped to dry it up and to heal it to various extents.

While a range of laser systems were discussed, I eventually decided to buy a low-level Class 3B laser-pen system. Some lasers have heads like a shower nozzle, designed to treat a wide area, but the laser pen is focussed, allowing treatment of specific acupuncture points. It is also very portable, and because it uses less energy there are fewer health and safety regulations. The laser light energy penetrates the skin and muscle to a known depth. The power, or dose rate, depends on the selected wavelength and length of time it is applied. The frequencies and programmes can be tailored to the type of tissue and condition.

I have heard people describe the various sensations they feel, which we can extrapolate to animals, and assume that they feel the same things. Sometimes there is no sensation, only that of the tip of the probe making contact with the skin. Or there may be a warm or radiating or pulsing feeling. Two people I treated described an unpleasant prickly sensation and asked for the power level to be reduced.

Husky Kiska was one of my first animal cases. She had a complex medical history but ultimately had been treated with acupuncture for spinal and tail pain at Glasgow Vet School. While overall she was more comfortable after each session, she was very dull and lethargic and took several days to recover. The laser option was discussed with the St Clair vets and Kiska came to me for acupuncture using the laser instead of needles. As you can see below, Kiska didn't mind!

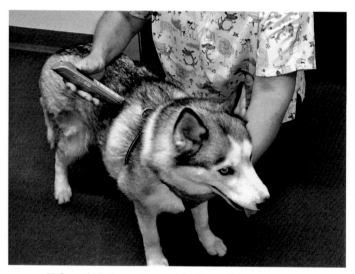

Kiska with the laser – too sensitive for needle acupuncture.

While people can understand that staying still during treatment is helpful, animals cannot. Old Spaniel Dylan was one of those! The tip of the laser pen has to be held next to the skin for several seconds so that the light energy is not absorbed by the fur, so a fidgety animal can be problematic. Vet Jenni and I still laugh at the pantomime that ensued while treating her dog, Dylan. Initially we used acupuncture to treat his sore back but sometimes Jenni (who was heavily pregnant at the time) struggled to restrain him from jumping off the table! Since the acupuncture was making a difference, we wanted to continue to treat him. Changing to laser made the sessions much easier.

Jenni later told me, "A combination of hydrotherapy initially, then acupuncture, really helped relax Dylan's muscles and kept him going for six months longer than I would have had him".

In general, laser therapy is well tolerated by both people and animals, which is illustrated by the following cases. Cob, Ellie and Mia are the most sensitive dogs I have come across.

Springer Spaniel Cob's hips and elbows

Cob joined the practice when he was ten years old. A few years before, he had condylar fractures in both his elbow joints, which had been repaired with screws. He was developing arthritis and had some joint rotation, which gave him a bandy-legged appearance and he sometimes stumbled. However, Cob was relatively unaware of all this. He was still chasing deer although it was all a bit more of an effort. His hind legs seemed to be slowing him more than his front legs. His owner John was hearing a clicking noise from somewhere in the hind leg area, so Cob was brought in for acupuncture.

We worked out that the click was coming from Cob's hips. He didn't like his front legs being touched, and would protest when I tried to treat his front half by wriggling and growling. It was just as well that his hips seemed to be the main issue. The aim was to slow down the rate of deterioration.

Regular acupuncture stopped the clicking in his hips and I also used points on his hind limbs to help his front limbs. Sometimes John would take the weight of Cob's head in his arms as Cob relaxed; on a couple of occasions he fell asleep and quietly snored! Cob improved and the improvement was maintained, but he had a big setback when he got lost in a forest, finally getting back home three hours later. John suspected he had run continuously for all that time, trying to find his way back. He took several days to recover.

Cob had acupuncture for two years until he began to need more treatment for his forelimbs. He was stumbling more often and slowing down. Any time I got near his shoulders or elbows he became growly, so I didn't pursue those points. It was a totally different matter with laser therapy. He still growled but nowhere near as often! He would come every four to six weeks for a top-up and his condition stabilised nicely.

Then one day, while on holiday, he suddenly became very staggery, his eyes flicked from side to side and he was sick. These were all the symptoms of the vestibular syndrome, a neurological condition in which balance is affected. He did recover, but not completely. His hind limb reflexes were slower and he had a wide-based stance as he tried to balance himself. His hips weren't clicking, but now it was becoming obvious that the vestibular condition was more of a threat to his well-being than his joints,

At Cob's last laser session he was very chilled out – he allowed me to treat his fore limbs and hind limbs and some head points in an attempt to help with the vestibular condition. He was still able to get in and out of the car although sometimes he wanted to be lifted. Unfortunately, the changes in his brain led to seizures from which he did not recover.

Ellie's spondylosis

Border Collie Ellie was not an easy patient. Her medical notes were dotted with comments about her nervousness, stating that she was grumbly and sometimes 'hyper'. She reacted any time she was touched and was always very tense, making it very difficult for any vet to carry out a meaningful orthopaedic assessment or manipulate her joints to find out if or where she was in pain.

However, at the age of ten, she was slower getting onto her hind legs and was scuffing her hind paws. Her vet Ian was able, after a few attempts, to pinpoint pain in her back. She was x-rayed and spondylosis in the lumbosacral area was found. Her mobility was helped by the anti-inflammatory meloxicam, but vet Ian and owner Carol decided she should have acupuncture and minimal medication.

With her history, I expected Ellie to be a challenge and, unlike Cob, knew she was never going to snore during treatment! I always try to use gentle restraint, but if Ellie wasn't going to cooperate perhaps acupuncture wouldn't be a viable option. At the first treatment she was noisy and managed to escape owner Carol's cuddle, jumping off the table after only four needles. But she did settle down again. She had shown some good twitch responses along her back.

At the second attempt she was even more vocal and jumped and yelped on a back point near the LS area – the site of her spondylosis. Before she came for her third treatment, she caught her left hind leg in a drain while out on a walk and cut her foot. She may have jarred her back at the same time because during treatment she responded with even more twitches. However, she was comfortable enough to let me massage her back after the acupuncture.

By the fourth treatment, completing her initial course, Carol said Ellie was behaving 'over the top', meaning that she was much more like her usual self! She was also scuffing her hind limbs less. We decided to try to treat Ellie on the floor on this occasion, and she was far less vocal and jumpy. We felt that there had been some progress and Carol and I could relax a bit.

By the next treatment, Carol described how playful Ellie had been – she had even pinched a tennis ball, which she hadn't done for some time, and Carol interpreted it as Ellie feeling so good that she was being naughty again! It seemed that the benefits of the treatment were lasting, so I increased the interval between appointments to six weeks and Carol only needed to use medication if there was some kind of setback, such as Ellie being bowled over by another dog.

Overall Ellie was less stiff and more active and playful, sometimes going without medication for two or three months, yet she was still unpredictable during her treatments. She would be totally settled but then let out a howl and start to fidget and jump, but often this wasn't related to a needle. This made her a good candidate for laser acupuncture. During treatments she was generally much calmer, with minimal reaction to the laser pen that I used at the same sites as the needles.

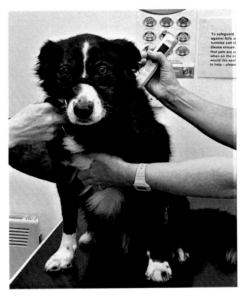

A settled Ellie during laser treatment.

Ellie also started physiotherapy, and received occasional medication until a bout of vomiting and diarrhoea led to a change of tablet. Galliprant™ (grapiprant) is a newer, different, albeit more expensive, class of non-steroidal anti-inflammatory drug that is given for pain and inflammation associated with osteoarthritis in dogs. Ellie had no side effects from it whatsoever.

At fourteen years of age, Ellie alternates between monthly laser and physiotherapy treatment and still gets in and out of the car well. Once, I didn't have my laser pen with me, so we tried needles again. She had the same jumpy reactions as before, confirming that she far preferred the laser!

Treating Mia's front limb, back and knee

In my experience, Rottweilers as a breed seem very sensitive to acupuncture. I regret that, before I had the laser pen, one Rottweiler I treated with acupuncture subsequently became wary of being examined in the show ring, because she was nervous of the treatment and therefore became suspicious about being handled. Hence, when Rottweiler Mia first came to me four years ago, it wasn't a surprise that she jumped when I inserted a needle. The location of the needle that made her jump differed every time and wasn't associated with a specific area of pain, but her owners Sharon and Nick knew that acupuncture was helping her.

Mia was lame on her left front leg and meloxicam and weight loss had been recommended. She had a lovely nature and happily jumped onto the table, never holding it against me when she reacted to a needle. In fact, she has remained one of my keenest patients, tugging at her lead in the waiting room to come into the room, and always giving me a hearty greeting – although now I do use the laser pen.

There was a six-month spell in which Mia was doing so well that she didn't need to have acupuncture. Then her left foreleg lameness returned. Arthritis was suspected in her elbows but she was more reactive to points on her spine at her next acupuncture session. Not long after, she had an emergency appointment when she was unable to use her hind legs properly and couldn't get in the car. Her owner Sharon had been hearing Mia's back 'crack', but it was thought that Mia had 'overdone' it while exercising, which had compounded the arthritis-related changes in her spine. With rest and increased medication, she made a good recovery.

After this, I extended Mia's acupuncture points along her spine to her pelvis. This elicited a huge yelp, several twitches and a bent needle, so I decided to use laser treatment. It seemed to be just as effective for her and she never had the same problem with her hind legs again. However, one day she ruptured the cruciate ligament in

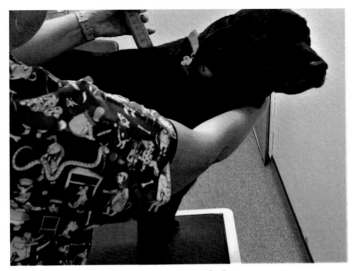

Mia was always happy to come for laser treatment.

her left knee, which required specialist surgery! Often when one cruciate has ruptured the other hind leg can be similarly affected, but so far all is well. She made a full recovery from the operation after three months of restricted exercise.

Without x-rays, it is now assumed that Mia has arthritis in several joints. She attends the clinic every two months for laser treatment, is on a half-dose of meloxicam, and she maintains an ideal weight. At eleven years old, she is still eager to come into the practice to see me and happily jumps onto the table (see below).

Recounting these experiences with the laser, I realise I still prefer to use needles. I feel there is more feedback from the body's reaction to needling, allowing problem areas to be better pinpointed. However, on occasion I do use laser acupuncture as a first choice and sometimes – with sensitive cases – I use it sooner than I once used to.

Jack Russell Terrier, Pip, is a more recent case (pictured *overpage*). She is much calmer with laser treatment than needles. Because of concerns with her kidney function, laser therapy is a safer option than medication and it helps with her mobility problems. She is still perky despite being seventeen years old, as you can see in the next photograph!

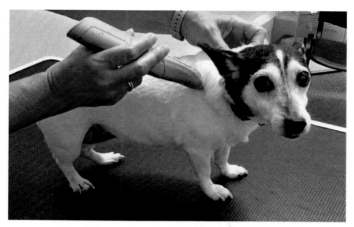

Pip aged seventeen – one of my oldest canine patients!.

Laser therapy is more popular nowadays for treating pain and reduced mobility. Some vets use it to target body areas, rather than acupuncture points. Of course, both animals and people are similar in the way they vary in their sensitivity to acupuncture, and some have more positive results than others. But there is one key difference – dogs and cats don't shed tears of emotion.

Diane's pain and anxiety

Diane's dog had a course of acupuncture some years before she called up about an appointment for herself. She had had a bout of shingles caused by the Herpes virus and was still in a lot of pain. She often felt muscular tension in her left shoulder, to which the shingles pain added, and she wondered if acupuncture could help. We decided to give it a go, but it was important that the skin around her shoulder had healed up, because the shingles blisters can contain the virus and we didn't want it to spread.

Diane said she had been feeling run down for a while, which may have contributed to her having shingles. She described her very busy life and the fact that she was constantly working to deadlines in her job. She exuded tension when I met her and I suspected she might be quite sensitive to acupuncture. I was quite taken aback by what happened.

With Diane lying comfortably on the couch, I chose small needles to minimise the dose of acupuncture and treated her ASAD points for pain and anxiety (Chapter 8). I explained that she may feel a bit emotional, but when I inserted the last needle, she said she felt a bit strange. Then she began to sob, uncontrollably. I quickly removed the needles. The treatment had released such a flood of emotions, to an extent I have rarely witnessed, that I suspected Diane needed to see her GP for another kind of help.

However, as Diane felt so much better regarding her pain and the way she felt in general after acupuncture, she wanted to continue, despite her overwhelming reaction. The next time I used even smaller needles and she was less tearful. We discussed the laser option and did use it on one occasion, but Diane didn't think it worked as well as the needles. She wanted to keep going with the treatments even after the shingles pain subsided. We progressed to include massage during her session, which eased the tension in her shoulders and added, as she described, to that 'feel-good factor'.

Diane had a lot of worries but she was holding it all together to reach particular work deadlines. She visited her GP and was signed off work to give her some time to recover. She still has regular top-ups of massage and acupuncture and has now started a new job and made other life changes.

In my experience, people like Diane who suffer with stress and anxiety benefit from this treatment. Some have been referred to me by a clinical psychologist who has a personal interest in massage and acupuncture; she knew that while she could help address the mental health issues of her patients, manual therapy could ease muscular tension which is often wrapped up with the anxiety or depression. It is well known that acupuncture can release emotions, but Diane's reaction was a memorable one!

There are continuous advances in laser technology and it is becoming more integrated into rehabilitation treatment for animals. Whether a laser or a needle is chosen depends on many factors, but laser is certainly handy for more sensitive people (Chapter 14) and feisty cats!

— 10 —

Feline ways

Dogs have masters – cats have staff!
Anonymous

Cats have been a constant presence in my life since childhood, and no doubt Tweak's accident contributed to my becoming a vet. While dogs far outnumber cats in veterinary practice and the majority of my veterinary acupuncture cases are canine, cats develop many of the same conditions as dogs, especially arthritic changes. They deserve their own chapter. In theory, even big cats, like snow leopards, could be treated with acupuncture – if they would let you!

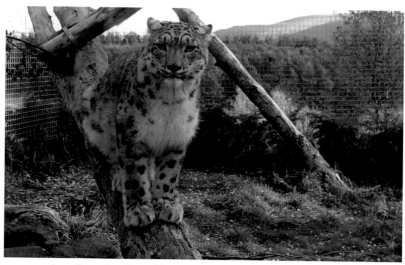

Snow leopard at the Highland Wildlife Park in Kincraig, near Aviemore.

They are simply different from dogs – a dog is more likely to do something to please. While overall cats are less predictable, they can still form the strongest of attachments to their owners. An exceptional example is Bob in the book *A Street Cat Named Bob* who shared his life with his chosen human (and author) James Bowen! Their special bond helped James overcome addiction.

Most people can't believe that our domestic cats can tolerate acupuncture. One of my earliest and most memorable cat cases was Lucky, a black cat who was certainly lucky and lived until he was nearly twenty-one.

Lucky and his type 2 diabetes mellitus

Owner Beth gave Lucky daily insulin injections and meticulously recorded his glucose urine levels. It's not an easy task collecting cats' urine but Lucky used a gravel-filled litter tray so a sample could be drained off and put in a bottle. Beth managed Lucky's diabetes extremely well, helping to maintain his glucose levels within the normal range. Beth understood the principals involved because she had type 2 diabetes herself, for which she took medication.

However, despite the best level of care, Lucky often had a sore mouth. He went off his food, became lethargic and had to be hospitalised when his blood glucose levels fluctuated. Cats with diabetes are notoriously trickier to stabilise than dogs, and it is difficult to predict how they will fare. Owner commitment is a major factor because there has to be a good routine in place for feeding times, insulin injections and observing their pet's drinking and urination. If their glucose levels are increased, for example, the pet may drink more and urinate more.

When vet Rachel asked me to treat eighteen-year-old Lucky's arthritic back and spine with acupuncture, I wasn't sure what I was taking on, or whether it would interfere with the diabetes control.

But Lucky was a good patient, and took to the acupuncture sessions just fine. His mobility improved and after starting acupuncture he was hospitalised less often – an interesting side effect! We gave up measuring his blood sugar levels as it didn't make sense to do it anymore. Why wasn't he comatose with the low levels he often had? Although there are far better tests available now, which give more accurate measures of sugar levels in the bloodstream, Lucky had such a good quality of life that we felt the least intervention possible was best for him. He never ceased to surprise me. If fact, he did so well that he ended up starring in an article in a cat magazine about my acupuncture clinic!

Lucky had been stable for a while when one day I had a call from Beth reporting that he was wandering around in circles. This didn't sound good and when he came to the practice, indeed he constantly circled to the left. There was no obvious problem with his ears, which can affect balance, and it was potentially very serious, likely indicating some central changes in his brain. Beth knew there may be no recovery but she asked if anything could be done – and especially what could acupuncture do? Using a steroid for potential inflammation in the brain couldn't be justified because it was contraindicated with diabetes, and as for acupuncture – well, I had no idea. I used my usual two points for any problem to do with the head. Lucky sat on the table, unbothered by the needles poking out from the skin between his ears and the back of his head. We decided to give him forty-eight hours following acupuncture, and if he was no better it would be best to put him to sleep.

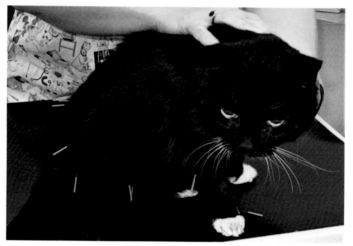

Acupuncture helped with more than diabetic Lucky's mobility!

I did not hear from Beth for a while and feared the worst when, at the appointed hour, she walked in carrying her basket and smiling. "Lucky's back to himself," she said. He lived for another fifteen months. Over that time he gradually became weaker until one day he couldn't get up.

Beth recalls how the practice boss had been at a conference where he spoke to a university expert about Lucky, telling her that it was most unusual for a cat to survive for nine years on treatment for diabetes. Lucky was certainly exceptional, but it has always left me wondering whether he would have lived as long were it not for acupuncture in the last three years of his life.

Amber and Katy—cats with very different personalities

In my experience, it's important to know how each cat reacts to being handled and to being groomed, and how they behave at the vets before considering acupuncture. My colleague Fiona, working at another branch of the practice, took the time to phone me rather than send the usual brief electronic message.

"I'm really not sure what you can do for Amber. Her owner has had laser treatment herself and thinks Amber would benefit. The trouble is Amber is a swiper! You never know when she's going to do it but she can lash out with her claws at the ready".

Oh no! All we could do was try. Despite medication, Amber was getting stiffer and finding it more difficult to climb stairs, so we considered it was worth trying laser acupuncture. Needles were completely out of the question. Cats are especially prone to kidney failure, which can be made worse by the use of some medications that Amber was already taking, and her latest kidney function test indicated signs of deterioration. If she tolerated the laser treatment it might be possible to use it to protect her kidneys, perhaps instead of medication, or at least with less.

On the day of Amber's first treatment, I tentatively removed the top half of the box she was in and saw her amber eyes looking up at me suspiciously. I turned the box round so she could see her owner Myra instead of me, at which point Myra moved her chair backwards, about

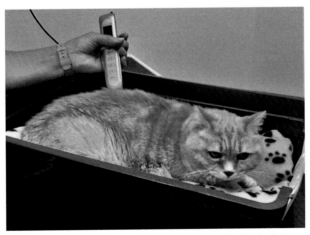

Amber could jump away at any time but stayed in her basket!

three feet away from the table. It dawned on me that this was so she was out of 'swiping distance' – a subtle warning of what might lie ahead!

We developed a method whereby I sat behind Amber, patting her head, while directing the probe of the laser pen into her fur, as close to the skin as possible, working at points up and down her back. I was alerted to any change of mood if her ears or tail started twitching, keeping my hand on her head so I could detect any movement – an early warning system! But Amber didn't swipe. When she got fed up, she occasionally hissed, and that signalled the end of her treatment. It was all on her terms. One day Amber surprised us. I thought I heard her purring, and Myra voiced the same opinion. She actually was – purring – and lovely as it was to hear it, I still couldn't trust her. We still kept her treatments to a minimum and, at the age of seventeen, she was much better at climbing the stairs and getting into her chair. The fact I managed to treat her while avoiding getting swiped highlighted that it's always worth trying treatment.

When Myra found that NHS laser treatment was no longer available for herself, for the chronic pain in her shoulder, she also came to me, at the GP clinic. She only needs a very short treatment, every three months or so, to keep the pain at bay.

Cats can be feisty, and there's no predicting how they will react and what they may or may not tolerate. When tabby cat Katy (pictured *opposite*) had acupuncture for her arthritis, it was a totally relaxing experience for all three of us – the cat, her owner and me. Her basket was already purring when she was brought into my room! She climbed out of her own accord and strutted around the table, allowing me to pet her. The whole process of coming for acupuncture was positive for Katy. It helped her mobility for quite some time, but the advanced arthritis in several of her leg joints made her more and more bandy-legged. At seventeen years of age, life became too much of a struggle for her.

Young Boris and Peggy—younger and very different too!

Boris and Peggy were younger cats with elbow problems. They had completely different experiences with acupuncture. Boris had an inflammatory type of joint disease affecting both of his elbows which was curtailing his activities. Treating him was always touch

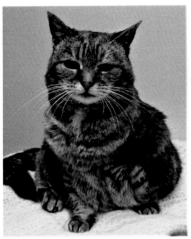
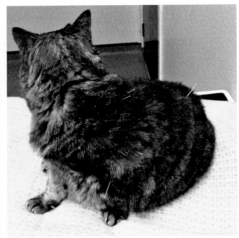

Katy was purring in these photos – even with the needles in place!

and go. He was always fidgety and could be pretty vocal during the session, but slowly he got used to the idea and eventually let me insert a couple of needles near his elbows. However, his behaviour changed dramatically during one particular visit. He came out of his basket in a very agitated and vocal state. I'd never seen him so angry. We worked out that it was because a Pointer puppy had recently joined the household, and for Boris coming to the vets for acupuncture was the last straw. Despite using a laser to minimise the interventions, Boris remained out of sorts and I had to abandon treatment.

Peggy was a dream. She was a Lilac Burmese with the loveliest soft fine grey fur. Acupuncture had been recommended to her owner Alastair

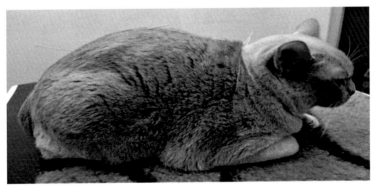

Peggy unfazed by the the needles that helped her to climb again.

by his regular vet, Fiona. Although Peggy was only seven years old, she had been diagnosed with arthritis in both elbows. X-rays had shown a typical furry appearance of her joints but luckily they were only early changes. She had been started on a course of anti-inflammatories the week before coming to see me, which had helped her, but at nearly five kilos she was a bit 'chunky'. The plan was to get her to lose weight at the same time as having acupuncture. Alastair was fully on board and decided to reduce her dry food. Peggy was sometimes lame on her left foreleg, even holding up her paw, and her whole demeanour changed. She was reluctant to jump either up or down, and couldn't get very far up her climbing frame, and bunny-hopped on the stairs. She was the ideal feline patient – always chilled out and purring, often lying on the table curled up on her blanket, and she loved to be stroked. She was completely unfazed by the needles; only if there was a tight area of muscle on her back or shoulder would she occasionally flinch or twitch.

It didn't take long for Peggy's normal behaviour to resume – mad half-hours running up and down the stairs, reaching the top of her climbing frame at full speed! She came for acupuncture every few weeks, and she lost weight and was on less medication. Alastair, who is a doctor, couldn't believe the transformation, and we've often discussed the potential of acupuncture in so many areas of medicine.

And the gorgeous Guinness

Here I must include my own cat – Guinness aka Guinny Boy. He came to us at the age of two (or three), via the Ryan and Calder practice where I was working in 2002. Guinness' owner was moving to a flat and was unable to take him. Having exhausted all re-homing possibilities, he thought the only option was to have him put to sleep. It was the last thing vet Aileen wanted to do so said she would try to find a home for him. It all coincided with Kenneth and I being cat-less; I had recently had to put our old cat Sumo to sleep, only six months after he had moved in. We were on holiday and on our return nurse Yvonne said there was a lovely big cat waiting for us. After spending two weeks in the practice, he had been truly 'vetted'; all the staff loved him so we had no qualms about adopting him. I had wondered whether he would be a handsome tabby or ginger but, as his name suggests, he was black and white.

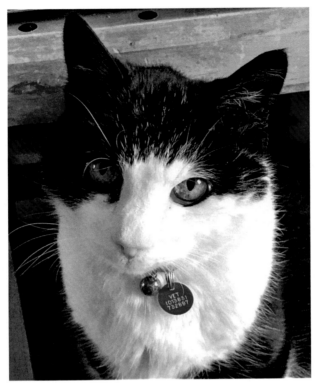

Guinness aged nineteen or twenty (I never knew his precise age).

Guinness had been neutered and well cared for and is one of that minority of cats who love their tummy being rubbed – a sure sign he had been handled often as a kitten and was good-natured. He turned out to be the friendliest of cats and wasn't averse to demanding attention. He was also boisterous – we thought someone was trying to break in the front door at first, but it was just Guinness, who had loosened the strip of draught excluder along the bottom of the door by pulling at it with his claws.

He has led a happy and uneventful life but as he sprawled out for a tummy rub one day, I found a small soft smooth lump near his groin. Guinness was unaware of it so I decided to just 'keep watch'. Sometime later a second lump appeared nearby, but this felt totally different, like a hard pea. He needed surgery to remove them. I never operated on him myself as I had stopped doing surgery by that time, so I was in the position of anxious owner! Decision made, vet Rachel operated. Much to our relief the lumps were both benign. I ignored the veterinary advice I would normally have given – to keep him inside for a couple of days. When we took Guinness home, he was so restless to go outside that I let him, with no untoward effects!

When a third fatty lump appeared on his side, I monitored it for a while until it grew bigger, so it was also removed. Pathology revealed it was also benign, just a fatty lump, but there was a chance of it recurring because it was attached to muscle and couldn't all be removed. The lump is still there, though it has reduced in size as Guinness has aged and lost weight.

Guinness later had some teeth removed when they became eroded near the gums. That didn't bother him either – the night after the operation he brought in a live mouse. At the same time, x-rays showed early arthritis in both his elbows; he had started to limp a little. He began to need some help around the age of fifteen, after I noticed him struggling to jump on the bed. I thought to myself that acupuncture was overdue and wondered what he would think of it. I tentatively began placing needles along his back as he lay relaxed on his side. To my surprise he continued to lie still as his coat quivered and twitched, as if there was an alien inside trying to burst out! Soon enough he was back to leaping onto the bed again with ease! Despite acupuncture, as he has aged he has become stiffer when getting up and down and sometimes limps on his left front leg.

Guinness was also diagnosed with a hyperactive thyroid gland, and a scan revealed an enlarged heart. He is maintained on tablets to regulate his thyroid-hormone levels and blood pressure alongside taking the anti-inflammatory meloxicam, and he also has acupuncture, of course, every now and then. At the age of nineteen (or twenty) he is a just a shadow of his former self but he still gets up and down the stairs to lie on the carpet above the hot water pipes, and he still purrs anytime he is touched or spoken to (sometimes you just need to look at him!). He truly is one of life's grateful cats.

— 11 —

Circling the dragons

Treating cats' elbows can be a challenge, but there is one relatively simple acupuncture technique that I have used time and again to treat a variety of 'dragons'

I had been taught about this traditional Chinese technique, known as circling the dragon while on both veterinary and human acupuncture courses. Needles are simply inserted into the skin in a circle around a problem area. It can heal lick granulomas in dogs, where they keep licking and chewing at their paw, for example, resulting in fur loss and red and sore skin, and it can promote healing of long-standing shin ulcers in elderly people. I had no idea what else it could do until a variety of cases presented themselves to me, where circling the dragon seemed appropriate. It produced some surprising results, as shown by the following three canine cases.

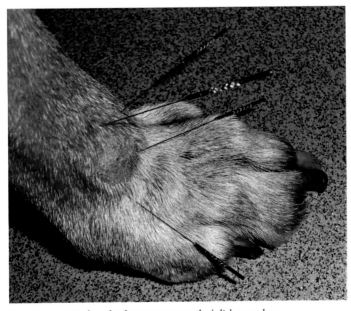

Circling the dragon to treat a dog's lick granuloma.

Oscar and Jamie's lumps

Oscar never stood still for long. A black Labrador of eight years of age, he was full of the joys of life and one of those older dogs that still had a pup inside. His owner Pat (from Chapter 3) was one of the first of my clients to try acupuncture for her pets. Oscar didn't just have arthritic hips, he also had liver problems and couldn't tolerate anti-inflammatories to help ease his pain. He had responded well to acupuncture and now just came for regular top-ups, but a growth had re-appeared on his right cheek, which I had previously removed surgically using a short-acting anaesthetic to protect his liver. Because of its location, below his right eye, the amount of tissue that could be removed was limited without more complicated and longer surgery, with an anaesthetic that wouldn't be good for him. I was disappointed to see it had regrown. No histopathology had been done under a microscope to determine whether the cells were benign or malignant because Pat did not want him to undergo any cancer treatment or major surgery.

As usual, he hurtled down the sloping corridor with his wide grin and tongue flopping, but I was surprised to see a plaster on his face. I removed it to reveal a seeping, ulcerated mass about four centimetres across. What a mess. Pat had put the plaster on in an attempt to stop her two other Labradors licking it. I felt we had to do something about it, but what?

During his top-up acupuncture treatment on the floor of my room, Pat and I discussed the issue. The mass was so unsightly it made people recoil, and now it was open and might get infected. Pat asked me what acupuncture might do. Nothing, I initially thought, but then I remembered the circling the dragon technique. I had never tried it for anything other than lick granulomas, but it had worked well for them. I hesitated.

"Well, I know the idea is if there is a red, fiery centre, circling it with needles can 'cool' it down."

But I couldn't reconcile this with my scientific training. Would it stimulate some form of healing in Oscar? Explaining this to Pat, I tried to open my mind to the possibility. I knew there was nothing to lose – and it certainly wouldn't do any harm. My doubting naysayer self never thought to take a photograph before I started to treat it.

Then there was the problem of inserting needles around the base of the growth so close to Oscar's eye. Would he let me? I didn't expect him to bite but you can never say never. I told Pat about Blue in Tasmania, the farm dog I was a stranger to who stood completely still and let me remove a piece of grass from his eye; and also about Scamp who had let me treat the cyst on his eyelid. In theory, Oscar was less of a challenge.

We lifted Oscar onto the table where Pat could hold him and give him a cuddle so he wouldn't take off round the room. I inserted a needle as close to the margin of the normal skin as possible, at the edge of the lump. It went amazingly well. Oscar allowed me to insert six needles to form a full circle and he didn't try once to paw at them or take them out.

So the procedure was acceptable to Oscar but I still wondered what it would achieve. The naysayer on my shoulder laughed loudly. But Pat had such faith that I didn't want her to be disappointed.

Next time I saw her was in passing and she called over to me, "I think there's a change, it's drying up!".

I was unable to disguise my scepticism, but when Oscar came for his next treatment, Pat was feeling pleased with herself.

"It's smaller," she pointed out.

I had to agree – possibly it was a little.

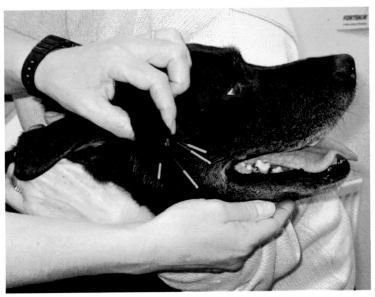

Oscar's reducing black growth circled with needles.

From then on, at each treatment session around four weeks apart, there was further improvement and no plaster was needed because the other dogs stopped licking it. Eventually the growth shrank from four centimetres to the size of half a thumbnail, now looking like a black tick. It rested snugly against his skin and its dark pigment meant it was hardly visible under his lovely thick black fur. Pat and I were both delighted and Pat was verging on smug. "See – I told you so!" she enthused. It felt truly humbling. I'd been taught a lesson by Pat and Oscar – to keep an open mind, to explore what acupuncture may do, and to give it a try even when my scientific brain was constantly questioning and saying, "Get a grip!".

One of my regrets is that we did not send the original sample away for pathology, because we had decided to avoid unnecessary expense. With such a good response to acupuncture it is probably safe to assume it was non-cancerous.

The lump never bothered Oscar (or tantalised his pals) again but another of Pat's dogs, chocolate Lab Jamie, developed a three-centimetre pendulous mass near his right elbow. He was totally unaware of it, but Pat pointed out that it looked awful and wondered what could be done about it. In fact, it looked like a testicle hanging from a thick neck of skin of about a centimetre across. I explained that the neck part was too wide to be tied off with suture thread to stop the rich blood supply to the growth, and hence shrink it. A general anaesthetic and surgical removal could not be justified for what was essentially a cosmetic procedure, although it would be justified if it prevented self-trauma that might result if it got caught on something. I wondered out loud to Pat – could acupuncture shrink the neck and then make it possible for it to be tied off? Of course she was a step ahead and had similar thoughts. I warned her that it could be unpleasant. If the blood supply was tied off the lump would probably swell up, go hard and discolour, plus there was a risk of infection. However, Pat's faith was – as always – unwavering.

Sure enough, after just a couple of sessions the neck shrank to half its size although the mass stayed the same. Then came the expectation for me to tie off the lump. It's an old-fashioned technique and I hadn't ligated a skin mass for a long time. There are other options these days, like cryo-units to freeze the tissue, and cautery to burn it off – but the lump was too big for these procedures. So I used catgut thread to wrap round the neck. Jamie barely reacted to the pressure of several knots being tied.

Two weeks later Pat laughed as she recounted recent events at home. Sure enough the lump had gone hard and discoloured, and was left dangling from Oscar's elbow. Pat's grandsons had been visiting and thought it looked disgusting. Then one day it had gone. She told me that the boys had great fun hunting the house and garden to find it, but they couldn't. The only gross conclusion was that Jamie – or one of his pals – had eaten it. Nevertheless, the skin healed perfectly and the lump never returned.

I told you about Izzy in Chapter 3 and Mia in Chapter 9. Like most dogs, they didn't mind their skin-lesion dragons being circled one little bit.

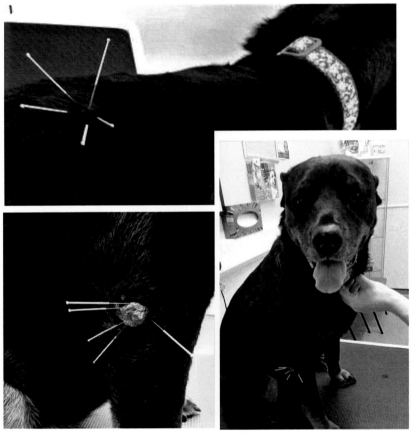

Circling a wart on Izzy's back and circling Mia's elbow.

Gabby's change of colour

Labrador cross Gabby had a different type of 'dragon'. She was stiff and her joints were visibly disfigured. She had been coming for acupuncture for a while to help her arthritic bandy legs. She was happier and more mobile on a maintenance routine of treatment every month or two. Unusually, she also had identical bald areas at the side of each knee, which never changed, and I had come to accept they were just there. I had never seen such symmetrical hair loss, both knees looking as if they had been shaved close to the skin in a circular patch approximately four centimetres in diameter. Owner Wilma was adamant that Gabby was not chewing the areas. This ruled out self-infliction which is sometimes due to irritated skin, or full anal glands, or a pain response. There was no thickened skin indicative of pressure sores, which are more often seen at the elbows anyway. The areas were simply bald and the only thing we couldn't rule out was that the hair loss was a side effect of her medication. In the past, steroid creams had been prescribed but had made no difference to the hair loss.

One day, I explained to Wilma about circling the dragon and how in some instances it stimulated healing. We considered what it might do for Gabby's bald patches. Gabby wasn't bothered about them at all, but I was intrigued as to why they were there. Usually when hair loss is

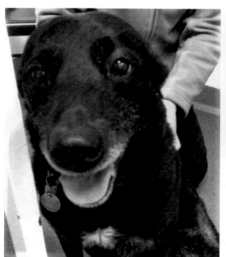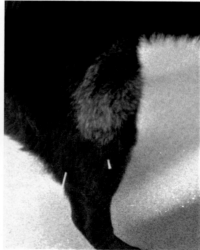

Gabby's white patch of fur just visible on her left knee and a close up of her right leg.

a side-effect of medication there is a more diffuse effect over the whole body, not just specific patches like the knees.

It helped that Gabby just loved coming for her sessions. Wilma said she was always excited when she realised where she was going. She would sit patiently in the waiting room, eyes fixed on my door as she waited for it to open. A few extra needles placed at the edges of the bald areas were fine by her and she never even noticed them as I circled both knees.

The next month, Gabby was back and we thought there was a little hair growth so we repeated the circling. By the second month there definitely was regrowth. There was no mistaking it. Her fur was coming back thickly, with the same normal texture as the rest of her fur, but white instead of black! Wilma was often stopped in the park by other dog walkers asking what had happened to Gabby's knees to cause the white spots. They, like Wilma and I, were surprised to hear that acupuncture had made her hair regrow!

I wondered what would happen as time went on. Would the hair loss recur? She was on the same medication, after all, and had had no more acupuncture at the site once her hair had come back. Well, the white patches of fur became peppered with black hairs, until eventually they were fully furred and black – just a few strands of white hair left to remind us where the changes had occurred.

We reached a stage where Gabby just needed acupuncture every two months to keep her condition as stable as possible, but then she started drinking more and began to lose weight. Blood tests revealed that her kidneys were failing. Gabby received acupuncture for three years until her failing kidneys took over.

It is important to point out that there are limitations to the use of acupuncture when it comes to circling the dragon. I was asked whether acupuncture could be used palliatively to treat a cancerous growth on Fly the Border Collie's paw. There was nothing to lose. Initially circling the area seemed to dry it up and the tissue around it became less inflamed. However, Fly had lost an alarming amount of weight when she came to her next session, and the next time she came the growth had mushroomed. The weight loss was an indicator of liver failure, which showed up on blood tests, and was probably due to internal spread of the tumour. Fly was beyond further treatment.

On another occasion, I used the technique for a troublesome cyst. Angel, a Samoyed, was prone to them forming in her skin and had already had several removed, and her owner Lynn was keen to avoid more surgery. Initially the cyst became smaller and drier, but later it enlarged and did need surgical removal.

Pat and her family moved south, but by then I had treated most of her pets – Labradors Oscar, Ishka, Ben and Dougal and her cat Suki – along with herself and her husband Paul. As she recalls, only Ben and Paul didn't have much response, however she had seen so many benefits that she considers acupuncture high on the list of treatment options for herself and others.

Now for three humans in whom I circled the dragon.

Gillian and Olivier's keloid scars

The success with Oscar's lump inspired me to try acupuncture for Gillian's scar. While I had been taught the circling technique could be used successfully to treat ulcers on the shins of elderly people, I wondered if keloid scarring would respond. I couldn't find any relevant information but the principle was the same – the needles would stimulate healthy tissue around the site to aid repair. Gillian's scar tissue on the inside of her left wrist, at the site of an earlier operation, was not just unsightly but painful. She was a veterinary nurse so she was constantly washing her hands and, because she had to wear short sleeves, the scar was exposed and prone to bumping and catching.

The scarring was the result of an accident some six months previously, when she'd been knocked over on an ice rink by a reckless skater. She had a Colles' fracture of the radius and ulna, the two bones in the forearm, close to the wrist. The fracture had been plated and had healed well but she had a keloid reaction where her body had overreacted to the healing process at the site of incision. The scar looked like a five-centimetre long, straight, fat red earthworm attached to her skin. Gillian had recently been told by her surgeon that her only option was plastic surgery, yet there was no guarantee that it would not produce another keloid scar.

She already knew how successful acupuncture had been in reducing the size of Oscar's lump so we talked about trying using the same technique for her scar. At her first treatment I inserted my smallest acupuncture needles (0.20 mm x 15 mm) a few millimetres deep and

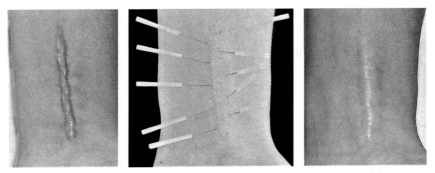

A keloid scar on Gillian's wrist at the first treatment (left); circling the dragon and the scar resolving (middle); after six months (right). This was published in the journal Acupuncture in Medicine *(Hunter, 2011).*

around a centimetre apart into Gillian's fine skin, circling the scar as close to the edge of the healthy tissue as possible. Sometimes I felt I had gone too near to the scar, when there was more resistance, at which point Gillian's face winced, but her arm never flinched and she kept still. Other than this, she felt little during the insertions, and there was just an occasional pinprick of blood. At the time she 'felt something happening' at the area overall but found it hard to describe – a slight feeling of heat, she ventured. The skin around the scar had tiny flat red spots, like a nettle sting but without the itchiness.

Fitting treatments in depended on Gillian's shifts and what time I had between my other patients, but over the next few weeks she came back and the scar began to shrink and became paler. After nine treatments over a four-month period the scar resolved significantly. It became painless, leaving only a pale, flat incision line. Needless to say, Gillian was delighted with the results and being able to avoid further surgery.

Sitting at home one snowy February day, I still hadn't heard of acupuncture being used for keloid scarring. I decided I should really do something with the series of photographs of Gillian's arm. The task of finding photos and cropping them and getting the wording right always takes longer than I expect, but I felt it was worth it in this case. I submitted before and after shots, with a short description of the process, to the BMAS journal, *Acupuncture in Medicine*, and was delighted when they were accepted for publication.

The photographs also went on display in the vet waiting room, where they happened to be seen by Catherine, the owner of Corton, an ageing wire-haired Dachshund with a squint pelvis and stiff back. Corton was coming to me on a regular basis for acupuncture which seemed to stop his mobility deteriorating and he was coping well. At his next session, Catherine quizzed me about keloid scars. Her husband Olivier had had heart surgery three years previously and a keloid scar had developed at the wound that ran down the middle of his chest. He had just been to his GP about the troublesome itch and had been referred to a dermatology consultant. He was offered steroid creams, which he'd had before, and there was no other treatment on offer. Catherine was excited to tell Olivier about the effect acupuncture had on Gillian's scar, but doubted whether he would go through with the treatment.

As it turned out, Olivier was more open to the process than we thought. He had seen Corton benefit from his treatments and duly arranged an appointment. Olivier had been born with a faulty heart valve, and cardiac surgery had repaired it; he had made a complete recovery and was fighting fit. Despite using various creams recommended by his doctor over the years, the protruding eight-inch scar down his sternum was still irritated by clothing, and he was very self-conscious about it when he swam or took his shirt off.

I expected that being such an old scar it would be too much of a challenge. Gillian's scar was only just six months old, but it had been three years since Olivier's surgery, and his scar was longer and thicker. My ever-present naysayer was casting doubt again.

Amazingly, after only one session of circling the dragon, the scar stopped itching against his clothing. Olivier was delighted even if that was all we achieved. I couldn't believe one treatment could be so effective and doubted it would last, but at the same time I thought of Gillian and the pale flat scar she'd been left with.

Olivier tolerated the needles perfectly well and, even when I hit a staple that had been left in place from the surgery, he said he felt it but it wasn't sore. Over several sessions, spaced out over the next year, the cord-like scar become flat and painless. In Olivier's words, "it deflated". Nowadays he has practically forgotten all about the pale scar on his chest.

As keloid scars are most common at incision sites at the wrist and sternum, and can persist indefinitely, I am aware that many people must be putting up with the associated pain, irritation and self-consciousness – and possibly could be helped by acupuncture. The needles may simply stimulate blood flow and various cells in the area to clean up and repair the damaged tissue. Of course, it's possible that some keloid scars repair spontaneously, but Gillian and Olivier didn't believe that was likely in their case. I believe that acupuncture could be offered for keloid scars in hospitals.

Because of my success with all these different animal and human 'dragons,' it is understandable that I felt confident enough to suggest treating one of my friends, another vet, with yet another type of 'dragon'.

A good look for James!

"What's that on your face?" I asked just after greeting a friend I hadn't seen for some months. I still cringe when I think how insensitive I must have sounded.

"Well, Jane, most people are not rude enough to ask!" came James's clipped response.

Oh no, my vet persona had surfaced and slipped out unhindered, but luckily James and I had been through vet school together. He was an 'F' and I was 'H' in the alphabetical register, so we had worked closely during our five years and had been good friends ever since. We could always take up where we left off.

I had never seen this unsightly swelling on the left side of his chin, though, sticking out from the edge of his clean-shaven jawline. James was such a particular person – his West End flat was like a show-house, and he was always immaculately groomed. This lump was so incongruous. It worried me.

"I'll tell you about it but let's get a table first."

He had travelled through from Glasgow to meet Kenneth and me at South Queensferry, a favourite childhood haunt of his. We were lunching in the Hawes Inn, of childhood importance to me too, although I'd never crossed the doorstep as a child. It was the special place where my bank-manager father had taken some of his customers (something you don't hear of these days). Now I occasionally go there for a meal and look out at the pier. The view always gives me a sense of satisfaction – a spectacular location at the base of the impressive Forth Rail Bridge, which was recently awarded World Heritage status. I always think about my swim across the strait of the Firth of Forth, a stretch of nearly one and a half miles, for which I trained for three years. Terrible conditions meant the swim had been cancelled two years in a row, but third time lucky – on the day of the swim the weather and sea conditions were so kind that my fellow swimmers and I – about thirty in total – all made it across.

On the day I was meeting James, the sun was shining across the river to Fife highlighting the Lomond Hills on the skyline. James told me his story. The red raised hairless one-centimetre lump had been there for several months and occasionally bled. It had started to appear when he was on a sun-soaked holiday in Mexico. As a sun-worshipper, he had been very worried it was UV-related and therefore possibly cancerous. His doctor referred him to a dermatology clinic. A cell sample was collected by fine needle biopsy, which involves inserting a needle into the mass and sucking up some cells into a syringe. Microscopy had revealed cells of an inflammatory origin – there was no sign of cancer – which meant his body was likely reacting to something and walling it off.

After James had endured the anxiety of wondering how serious it was, he now believed it was most probably down to an in-growing hair. I ticked off my mental check list: he was feeling well; he had been to his GP then saw a consultant; a diagnosis had been made through examining the tissue; he'd had a course of antibiotics in case of infection (which had no effect); nothing more could be done medically. His only option, therefore, was surgical removal, which could leave a scar.

Unless … I wondered if acupuncture could help. Perhaps, if nothing else, it would make it smaller so the surgery would be easier, with less scarring. What would James think of the suggestion? Kenneth knew what was coming.

"So, do you want me to 'circle your dragon'?"

James burst out laughing.

I had a smile on my face as I explained, to the best of my ability, what traditional Chinese acupuncturists mean by circling the dragon, with its fiery red centre and needles circling around its base to cool it down – a totally different way of looking at it from Western medicine, where it was considered to be an inflammatory process. So I told him about some cases I'd treated successfully, with lesions that fitted the 'dragon' description – Oscar, Jamie, Olivier and Gillian sprang instantly to mind although their 'dragons' were different from his. If it were me, I'd give it a go, I told him.

"Jane, I'll try anything!" he said.

We arranged for him to come to the clinic. He didn't move as I tapped six needles in place, as close to the base of the lump as I could. I suggested that one treatment may not do much and that he should find a local practitioner in Glasgow for follow-up treatments. Of course that didn't happen and a few months later, I went to a course in Glasgow and stayed overnight at James' home – the lump was still there. Apparently, it had started to get a little smaller but then resumed its usual size. He was happy to try another treatment, so that evening in his flat I needled deeper around the base. Again, I suggested follow-up treatment with someone local and again several months passed.

The next time we met, I looked for the lump straight away.

"What is it?" he said, frowning at me.

"James, have you had surgery?" I asked, searching his face for a tell-tale scar.

"No, I didn't. Didn't I tell you? You made it go away!"

I looked closer. No scar. We shared our amazement. Two vet degrees and a PhD each and we were astounded at what a few small needles could achieve. Circling the dragon had worked again!

'Well, Jane. I'd rather think that you simply activated my macrophages,' he continued with a laugh as we reflected on our body's amazing ability to heal.

For many years, James was a researcher in immunology (the science of how our bodies recognise and eliminate foreign particles, including bacteria and viruses that may be harmful to us). He is used to analysing 'evidence' and has published many scientific papers. He considers that acupuncture triggered an inflammatory response – stimulating macrophages in particular; they're the cells that scavenge and take up the debris from pathogens and dead cells, which had a healing effect in this instance. James is very glad of the outcome and agrees it is a treatment option that should be further explored.

The following two cases of a dog and her owner show when it is worth at least *trying* acupuncture when conventional treatment hasn't resolved a condition.

— 12 —

Acupuncture improves a dog's behaviour—and her owner's foot!

Peanut was a case referred from the Glasgow vet school and her notes made complicated reading! She was considered a 'behavioural case' and had already been seen by Sam Lindley, a vet who specialises in behaviour and pain cases and an experienced veterinary acupuncturist who runs the school's pain clinic. Sam also lectures for BMAS and, in addition, as part of the Western Veterinary Acupuncture Group, has taught foundation acupuncture courses to vets and nurses since 2000.

Peanut was an eight-year-old yellow Labrador whose bouts of destructive behaviour were of great concern to owners Aleks and Bryan, two busy young parents, one of whom ran a dental practice while the other was an accountant, with two young children and a third on the way! Sam had finally worked out that Peanut's problems were due to the clicking sound of the central heating switching on and off – she had conditioned herself to think it was the cause of her back pain! This sounded a bit bizarre to me, but after a full investigation at the vet school, her back pain was considered to be the underlying cause of her behaviour problems. As Peanut only lived six miles from Dunfermline, she was referred to me by Sam and a neighbouring veterinary practice to continue her treatment instead of having to travel all the way to Glasgow. This sounded like one crazy dog!

Sam had included a list of Peanut's needle points but warned me that Peanut was very sensitive to acupuncture. Not many needles were needed to make her very sleepy. The plan was to insert needles along either side of her spine so then she could lie down and relax while they did their job. She was an ideal patient because she had been thoroughly investigated and had already been responding to acupuncture.

Peanut had been very unsettled at night despite being on gabapentin for her pain. I included the same points as Sam but added a few more, getting a yelp at a pelvic point and a reaction at knee points, along with lumbar twitches. Peanut was indeed sensitive to acupuncture and it was obvious how much brighter and skippier she was after her sessions. Over the next few treatments she eventually lay down and relaxed, and her mobility improved overall but there were ups and downs; she was prone to having anxious, restless nights and couldn't be trusted not to cause damage in the house when everyone was asleep. Sometimes she had better nights when she slept in Aleks and Bryan's garage. Sometimes she needed a diazepam sedative tablet, but not so often with the acupuncture. Her behaviour kept improving and over time her treatment settled down to six-week intervals, which seemed to work well for her and Aleks could tell when she needed a top-up.

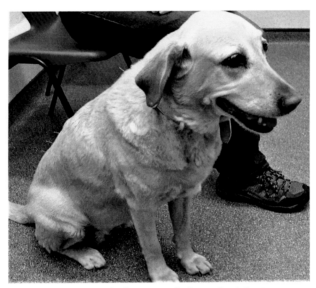

Peanut – pain had an unusual effect on her behaviour.

It was usually Aleks who brought Peanut into the clinic, but Bryan had attended the last few appointments. As I worked with the needles, I explained to Bryan in more detail about treating Peanuts' BL11 points between the shoulder blades (the Bladder points on a traditional Chinese body map) to help her arthritis specifically. Bryan later told me it was this discussion, about arthritis, that prompted him to tell his own story.

He had just got back after two weeks at Disney World and was feeling miserable about his feet. They were sore – walking around with his wife and young family had been torture. He was devastated when his sore feet and blood results indicated the likelihood of rheumatoid arthritis, especially about what that meant in the long term. Although his consultant couldn't be certain about the diagnosis, it all added up and Bryan was initially prescribed methotrexate. However, it can affect the liver and he wasn't allowed to drink alcohol. It also made his eczema worse. While his feet had become less painful, he then had to stop the drug because his liver enzymes climbed above normal, indicating some degree of liver damage.

He still couldn't run and even had to wear trainers when he went to the Edinburgh accountancy firm where he worked. It was having a great impact on his life. However, he told me he had had surgery on both feet about a year ago for Morton's neuroma, in which painful nodules form around a nerve. I wondered whether there might be some lasting post-operative effect which was confusing the picture. Could massage and acupuncture help? So I asked him if he would consider it. Yes, he said, he would, but who could treat him? He didn't know that I also treat people …

After getting permission from his consultant – who felt it would do no harm while not expecting it to do any good – we started to explore what manual therapy would do. The difficulty was that Bryan was very apprehensive and had very sensitive feet – which was quite evident when I first started to massage them! I explained the massage was a good way to pinpoint swelling and pain. Both of his feet were swollen around the ball, and the left foot was swollen over the metatarsals (the long bones in the foot that footballers sometimes break) and some areas were very sore to touch! However the pain was localised, all around the scars from his operation sites – not at the joints. My fingers felt a crunching sensation around the scar on his left foot and Bryan reacted even more. Then came the acupuncture. I used my smallest needles but he was very sensitive between his toes, and reacted more than a lot of dogs do. Peanut had been an easier patient by far!

At the next treatment, Bryan reported that he'd already felt an improvement and had been able to walk to work at a good pace in his trainers. There was less swelling across the metatarsals, but the soles at the balls of his feet were thickened. Similar points were needled again because now Bryan was willing to put up with anything that helped.

At his next visit Bryan had been doing a lot of walking and had sore shins as a result! The left metatarsal area was swollen, especially around the middle toe and sole underneath. Bryan said that at its worst the toes on either side of the operation site felt achy, and the pain shifted around, but he had managed to walk more. I thought that strengthening the treatment with electro-acupuncture at the operation site could be of further help, and may stimulate further healing, especially as he was so keen to do more activities. I attached the crocodile clips between the two needles and adjusted the current according to what Bryan was feeling.

Unfortunately, Bryan did not have a good week after that electro-acupuncture session; he had three painful episodes in a single day so it was abandoned! Next came laser treatment using a 3B laser pen. When against the skin the light beam can penetrate skin and muscle to reach the acupuncture points. The same sites I used with needles were each treated for twenty to thirty seconds, and I could also treat points on the soles of his feet without the discomfort of needling.

This was the best form of treatment for Bryan and so we continued to use it. After the initial course of four sessions, we were able to increase the interval between them to four and then six weeks as he improved. At his sixth treatment Bryan was aware of pain across the metatarsals, with the right foot being sorer than the left. On massage, he was very sore with deep pressure at the operation site on that foot, describing it as the worst pain he'd had since the first massage. However, at his next visit Bryan reported that he hadn't had any discomfort on a regular basis. The metatarsal pain had gone, leaving only the odd twinge when sitting at work, and in the last three weeks there had been no pain at all.

This went on for another two months, but Bryan went out road running, causing pain in his shins and base of his left big toe. The following day he came for massage. There was no crunching in his left foot but there was mild discomfort on pressure at the end of both operation sites. Another two months later and, at what turned out to be the last appointment for a preventive laser treatment, Bryan had no foot pain and had even been discharged by his consultant.

The last time Bryan came along with Peanut he had just returned with the family from another two-week Disney holiday. He reminded me that it was five years since the last one, when he'd been grumpy and in pain and walking was a daily chore. This time he said his family couldn't keep up with him (and he was also able to enjoy a glass of beer or wine!). His consultant couldn't explain the improvement from acupuncture and said he expects the rheumatoid arthritis to appear in the future, but Bryan's feet are still pain-free and whatever the future holds, for five years he has managed to avoid medication that would have had a detrimental effect on his liver – yet another lesson to me, that it is worth seeing what massage and acupuncture can do to help in situations that are new to me.

Meanwhile, Peanut is in her seventh year of acupuncture. Ageing and deafness have no doubt contributed to her mellower and calmer character. She doesn't walk very far and just does as much exercise as she feels like. She has recently been diagnosed with a liver complaint but is still coping well. Aleks and Bryan feel that, at over fourteen years of age, she is still enjoying life, and they attribute much of her well-being to acupuncture. Bryan is a wonderful advocate of acupuncture after his and Peanut's experiences but he is adamant that he prefers laser to needles!

The 'square' spaniel and other weighty stories

If we could give every individual the right amount of nourishment and exercise, not too little and not too much, we would have found the safest way to health.—Hippocrates

It was the first time Shona and I had arranged to swim together, some last-minute training at Aberdour for another River Forth swim. The calm sea and lovely sunshine were giving the impression that the water was going to be warm rather than 'baltic'. As we got changed, Pickles, Shona and partner Chris's Lhasa Apso were scouting about further along the beach. Chris was in charge as Shona and I headed for the sea. It's not often I meet a patient outside of work but Pickles had spotted us and came tearing towards us. She ignored Shona and surprisingly came straight to me. I suspected she remembered all the treats I'd given her over the past two years at the clinic. The wetsuit I was wearing didn't make any difference to her, but with no treats to hand I just made a fuss of her. It was so lovely to see her in action like that. Her once sedentary life had been transformed with acupuncture and weight loss.

I recently looked back at her history. I'd first seen Pickles when she was only seven weeks old for her first check up and vaccination. Shona's sister's Lhasa Apso had had pups and Pickles was their pick of the litter. As she lay on her tummy on the table, she could have been mistaken for a long-haired guinea pig – just a small ball of fur. It was hard to tell the nose end from the tail end! It would be over four years before our paths crossed again, but in those years Pickles had been a frequent visitor to the vets.

At four months old she was checked over after twisting the lead round her legs and falling downstairs, hurting one of her hind legs. Not long after, she had fun bull-dozing the sand on the beach with her face, and eating seaweed. She began vomiting and on examination a hard loop of bowel was felt in her abdomen. When she was x-rayed for a suspected blockage, her colon or large bowel was found to be full of sand. She had been eating the sand – not just playing with it! Luckily, her intestines were still working and lots of sand eventually appeared from the other end with no damage done.

Her neutering had to be postponed because of a false pregnancy, and another time she was brought in because she'd begun to hop occasionally on her right hind leg. Another x-ray and specialist opinion later and it seemed that her patellae (kneecaps) were slipping in and out of the groove they should lie in, but she had no pain. This is a common finding in short-legged breeds like Lhasa Apsos, and usually nothing needs to be done unless it becomes a more serious problem. In Pickles' second year she had episodes of being lethargic, puffing and panting, with intermittent vomiting and a possibly a sore back. Further x-rays followed, of her chest, and she was tested and found negative for lungworm, which is an unusual diagnosis in the UK but something we need to watch out for. Her heart was monitored too, but nothing significant was found. Her neutering went well but she was still vomiting every two weeks or so for no apparent reason. An antacid was prescribed and it seemed to help, so it was thought the vomiting may have been linked to her being anxious and upset by loud noises. She cried sometimes, and could be anti-social; sometimes she was lethargic and wasn't keen on walks.

All in all, it was a very confusing picture but Chris and Shona wanted to find out more, so when she was four and a half, the practice referred Pickles to the behaviour and pain clinic at the Glasgow vet school to see Sam Lindley who had also seen Peanut (Chapter 12). At the end of her assessment, Sam believed Pickles was reacting mostly to pain; while her legs seemed comfortable despite both kneecaps slipping, she had chronic back pain. Three pain medications were prescribed and further investigations were recommended. Back at her own vet's practice she was re-examined, but nothing abnormal was found on x-rays of her spine, pelvis or knees. She had been making some louder-than-normal 'piglet' noises so her throat was examined while she was under anaesthetic, which revealed an excess of soft tissue. This is typical of her breed but weighing-in at ten kilograms – around two kilos overweight – was not helping her. Lhasa Apsos have a small body with short legs and a long back – like Dachshunds, which are notorious for spinal problems especially with the strain of extra weight.

Although the spinal x-rays were clear, Chris and Shona were still worried because of what had happened to Pickles' brother. He'd had surgery on two occasions to remove prolapsed discs which had caused him to be 'off his legs' and in a lot of pain. Although he seemed to recover well, it happened a third time when he was older; this time it was considered too much to put him through another operation so he was put to sleep. Their fear of this happening to Pickles was understandable.

To rule out a spinal cord problem an MRI scan was carried out. An x-ray only shows bony changes and because discs are made from a jelly-like substance they only show up if they are calcified (hardened). The MRI results, however, were normal – no bulging discs or stenosis (narrowing) of the spinal canal. But multiple discs were dehydrated and degenerated, also common in Lhasa Apsos, and there was no indication for surgery. However, she did have significant pain in the lower back. Along with her medicines, acupuncture was recommended and Pickles was referred to me. It was hoped that most of her problem was muscular and that acupuncture would help, so four and a half years later a mature Pickles arrived at my door.

She had already improved on a high dose of six pain-killing gabapentin tablets every day, plus intermittent doses of the liquid anti-inflammatory meloxicam. She had minimal exercise and this was closely managed by Chris and Shona. Life for Pickles wasn't much fun.

I heard Pickles coming long before I saw her. She began barking as soon as she got into the waiting room. She was always very vocal – it was her trademark. She continued barking as I approached her, quite a big noise for such a small dog, and I wondered how the acupuncture would go as she eyed me suspiciously. She walked well, following Chris and Shona into the room, and much to their surprise was actually very relaxed through her first session.

I concentrated on treating her back. The muscles in the mid-back area felt tight on needling, which resulted in good twitches. She yawned – a good sign that the acupuncture was stimulating the release of feel-good hormones and making her a bit tired. I suggested reducing her tablets straight away as I was very hopeful that if we could release her tight muscles the pain would reduce and her mobility improve. After two sessions she was managing to walk round the shore of the local loch again, and was comfortable on reduced medication. By the fourth session, the gabapentin and meloxicam doses she had been on for three months were halved, and Pickles was doing even better – running and happy. However, she sometimes hopped on her right hind leg, so I included points specific for her knees and continued to see her monthly.

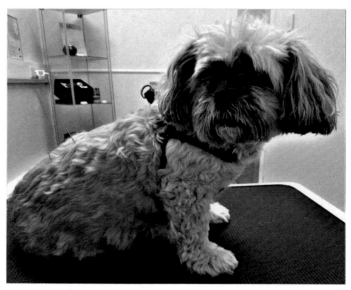

Pickles during acupuncture – needles visible on her back.

Occasionally she gave a yip at needles in her right or left knee points, and once I didn't treat her knees at all because she snapped at me during her back treatment.

Sessions varied quite a bit with Pickles, and when she'd been limping on a front leg I wondered what was up. Luckily it was nothing sinister, just hard compacted fur and muck wedged behind her toes. She really had been having a good time out and about!

Despite the marked improvement and being on only one gabapentin tablet a day, nine months into her acupuncture I didn't think that Pickles was at her best. She still weighed around ten kilos and had no 'waist'. She had been around two kilos overweight for a while, and Chris and Shona had tried to reduce her weight, without success, but I knew the best outlook for her would be if she weighed less and had less pressure on her long back and little short legs.

The problem was that her owners felt they just couldn't feed her any less, so during that first year of acupuncture she stayed around the ten-kilogram mark. They were so pleased about how well she was doing, so there was little motivation to work on her diet. However, as Chris reminds me, it was the story I told them about a certain Spaniel that inspired them to try again.

It can be hard for owners to take on board the importance of weight loss. Obesity is very prevalent and can increase the risk of disease, impair movement, shorten lifespan and overall reduce quality of life – just as it does in humans. Whether obesity should be classed as a 'disease' is debated by both the veterinary and medical professions, but it's part of every vet's duty of care to give appropriate advice. To this end, I often speak about Ted – the 'square Spaniel' – which is a very surprising weight-loss tale.

Nurses Kelly and Sandra knew I would readily tackle a pet's weight problem with an owner, but for the next appointment I was advised not to say anything because it would be a complete waste of time. Kelly and Sandra had both been in the small branch surgery for many years and knew the owners and their pets so well that their experience was often invaluable; they would also give excellent supportive advice on weight loss and behaviour problems. Sandra was very embarrassed once, when her knowledge of treats and bad behaviour backfired on her. Out with her small daughter, Brooke, one day, they passed a mother with a young boy in the throes of a tantrum. The mother gave him a bar of chocolate to quiet him down. Brooke commented in a surprised and very loud voice, "Mummy, why is that boy being rewarded for bad behaviour?". Out of the mouth of babes, they say. Growing up in a household with two Rottweilers, of which Sandra had good control, Brooke was noticing the similarity between some dog and child behaviours.

Back to Ted, the square spaniel. His owner had been given the best of advice many times over and had bought the expensive special-diet food for Ted, but Ted just got bigger. Where his waist should be he actually looked square! He had a big belly and the fat pads in front of the pelvis made it look like he had a square saddle round his middle. It was with great difficulty that I didn't mention his size as I dutifully went through the routine consultation, with examination and annual vaccination. However, Ted's owner confided that the spaniel wasn't coping well with the stairs of their first-floor flat, taking his time, and generally being a bit slower. Otherwise he was fine, and there certainly wasn't anything wrong with his appetite. But Ted's owner was worried. He said he'd expected to get a row about Ted's weight, so I decided to go for it. After all, he had brought up the subject – not me.

"Well, as we get older, we can slow up and get stiffer," I said, "but the best thing you can do for Ted is weight loss." I knew he had heard it all before, but I went on to explain that Ted's slowness and difficulty climbing stairs was because he was carrying the equivalent of a three- or four-kilo rucksack. I could feel a change in the owner. Keeping things simple, I said, and feeding him less dry food and more tuna and carrots could be helpful. I left it at that. Carrots are so low in calories. despite looking bulky, and are a good filler, but they should be given in small enough pieces not to cause choking. We arranged for Ted to come back for a weight check with the nurses and to see me in a month's time.

Six weeks went by until Ted next came to see me and what a change! His owner was delighted. Ted no longer had a problem going up and down the stairs, and was enjoying running around in their park. It was as if he had lost several years in age, never mind in weight! And what a weight loss! Almost too much, in fact – nearly three kilograms in a very short time.

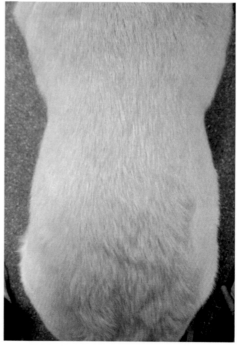

Kola's hourglass waist – head end at the top!

Ted's owner said he had done as I suggested, just feeding him tuna and carrots. Oh no! He had misheard me and completely cut out his standard dog food! I didn't have the heart to tell him he had made a mistake, but I did say that now was the time to reintroduce complete meals. I fully expected Ted to pile on the weight again as it would be trial and error to get the amount right, but one month later his weight was the same. I had to reassure the disappointed owner – it was fine that Ted had not lost any more weight; he had found just the right amount to feed him and should just keep doing what he was doing to maintain his new lower weight. I was pleased for both of them that we'd found a solution to Ted being slow, and square. He had a waist again, and was zipping around once more. The owner was delighted he had a fitter rejuvenated pal.

As a guide, when we look down on a dog from above, their body should have an hourglass shape; from the side their outline should be like that of a greyhound – a tucked-up abdomen and defined waist. Someone once said to me that some breeds of dog don't have a waist, but they all should! It is just that too many are overweight and our perception has changed. The ideal body shape is illustrated by Kola and there are body condition score charts available, which show pictures of the ideal shapes of both cats and dogs. The one illustrated *overpage* (Fig. 9) is produced by the World Small Animal Veterinary Association (WSAVA).

The importance of diet cannot be underestimated. Dogs have a carnivorous bias to their diet and lots of research has gone into producing processed dog foods that create a balanced diet. I have seen an extreme case of rickets in a Hungarian Vizsla puppy who was brought to me, one Hogmanay, because she was unable to stand on her hind legs. She had fractures in both of them. Luckily, I was able to refer her to the specialist orthopaedic clinic for repair. They confirmed she had 'folding' fractures of the femur (equivalent to our thighs) in both back legs because she was on a home-made diet of mince and rice – as recommended by her breeder. But the lack of calcium had weakened her bones. Dogs can also digest carbohydrate-based foods because they are omnivores, meaning they can eat both meat and vegetables. Owners often do not know that vegetables can form part of their dog's diet. 'Tuna and carrots' is not a good long-term diet but it served a purpose for Ted.

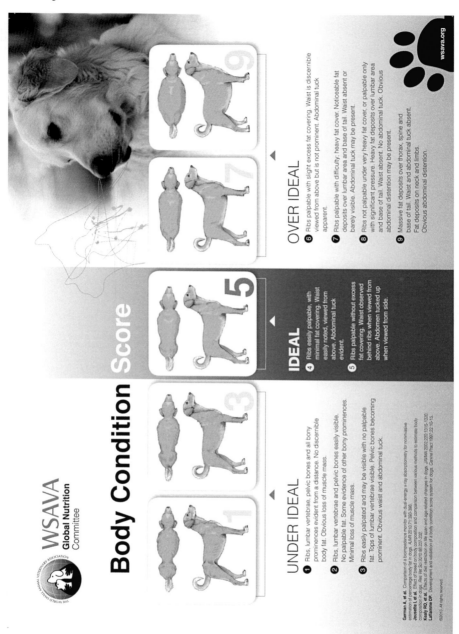

Fig. 9: The World Small Animal Veterinary Association's (WSAVA) body condition score chart, describing the appearance of a dog with an ideal weight and body score of 5, compared to being underweight or overweight. It is available at http://www.wsava.org/nutrition-toolkit.

On hearing Ted's story, Chris and Shona decided to make another big effort with Pickles, to try her on veggies, which is when a very satisfying change occurred. Her weight began to steadily decrease, slowly at first and then more markedly. The solution had been to replace her biscuit treats with red peppers – she loved them! Pickles eventually lost the extra two kilos, coming down to eight kilos, equivalent to a loss of twenty per cent of her bodyweight. This is a massively significant weight loss for a small dog. At a talk by Dylan Clements, an orthopaedic specialist at the Dick vet school in Edinburgh, weight loss was at the top of his list when it came to treatment of mobility problems and osteoarthritis in dogs. Around five per cent of dogs have a visible change in lameness, and in ten per cent changes can be seen when they walk on a pressure plate, which records weight distribution.

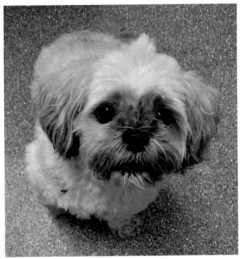

Pickles waiting for a treat after acupuncture!.

Two years on, Pickles still has maintenance acupuncture every six to eight weeks. After twenty long months of medication she now needs none and her weight is maintained at around eight kilograms. Occasionally her eyes need a wipe but at her recent routine health check vet Sandra noted no complaints. Miss Pickles, as she nicknamed her, was doing very well. She can tear up and down the beach with her only medication being a sedative, a tablet of diazepam, once a year in November because of her fear of fireworks. Then she can watch them without being scared!

Another weight-loss success story is Kara's, which may also have been inspired by Ted's experience. I smile when I think of her and the surprise discovery by her owners, Joe and Carol, of a certain healthy food option! Cavalier King Charles Spaniel Kara had been referred because of her knee and back. However, her history also included details of a heart problem. A year before coming to me, she had been diagnosed with a heart murmur but had no clinical signs such as coughing or lethargy. She had been admitted for x-rays, which revealed spondylosis due to arthritic changes around the vertebrae. It was only mild at L2/3 with more at L7/S1, but more significantly she had a partial rupture of the cruciate ligament of her right knee, requiring surgery to stabilise it.

Then her heart murmur worsened and started to affect her breathing. She needed a diuretic to get rid of fluid build-up in her lungs as well as her usual heart medication. And she also had a sore back. She was tentative when walking, with her back slightly hunched, and that is what prompted vet Emma to suggest acupuncture.

Kara was on several tablets, both for her heart and for pain control, and had been doing quite well when I first saw her. She was swimming sometimes and more active and not stumbling as much on her foreleg when she went up or down steps. I started treating her back and got good lumbar twitch responses, indicating that her muscles were tight. Kara was also overweight – by a lot. She was small for a Cavalier, but very round. I thought how much her heart would benefit if it had less weight to cope with, as would her knees and back. Looking at her chart I saw she had been seven or eight kilos around three years ago. Now she was heading towards eleven, despite being on a special dry diet dog food for weight loss!

I knew other vets would have already advised that it was best for Kara to lose weight and I feared that there was no point in me going over it again. Kara's owners were seeking help from acupuncture because they wanted to do the best for her, yet I felt my hands were tied. Weight loss along with the acupuncture could be amazing, just as it was for Pickles, and after the success with Ted I had at least to try.

I asked about Kara's feeding regimen. Her diet dog food was measured out, but owner Joe explained that his wife Carol fed Kara from the table and he didn't see how that could change. It conjured up an image of my father sitting at the dining table when my parents had two Cavaliers. Roy was heavier than Sandy, largely because Roy was ever-present at the table, just sitting there gazing adoringly at Dad with those big Spaniel eyes, waiting on titbits. When I challenged Dad about feeding Roy from the table, and pointed out that thickly buttered oatcakes sometimes with 'just a wee piece of cheese' were not helping his waistline, he got very defensive. It is often a joy to feed our pets and it can be very difficult to curtail our habits, so weight and feeding are very sensitive subjects.

To my shame, I recall when, as a new graduate at the end of a very tiring day, I was presented with an extremely overweight Old English Sheepdog for examination. I said, "Hello fatty"! I can still see the look of hurt on the owner's face as she replied, "She's not fat – she's fluffy!". While we never want to upset owners by being too critical, it is challenging to find a manageable way forward. Feeding our pets is linked to kindness, and when we are told that feeding them less is better it can be interpreted as being unkind. It isn't surprising that advice often fails. The fact that some dogs, especially Labradors, seem to have a bottomless pit for a stomach means there is no satisfying them; they are always seeking more food and have ways and means of enticing their owners to comply with their demands. It can be a real mind-game!

"Perhaps Kara's routine doesn't need to change if we can find something low calorie that she will like?" I suggested, mentioning the possibility of a vegetable treat. The fact that Kara wasn't fussy and ate everything would come in very handy.

At the second acupuncture session I was astounded to see that Kara had lost almost a kilogram. This time it was bags of diced carrots and swedes! Kara simply loved them, partly cooked or raw, and would even root through the vegetable basket for carrots. The trick was working well, but almost too well – that was a lot of weight to lose in just one week. Again Kara had a good response to the acupuncture. She had also been rolling on her back and wanting her tummy rubbed, which she hadn't done for months, so was already feeling better. By the fourth treatment, she was going for longer walks and she didn't whimper when her hind legs were manipulated. At her fifth treatment, six weeks after we started, Kara had a definite waist, and at seven-and-a-half kilos (nearly three kilos down) it was time to stop her special diet and get back to regular dog food. There were minimal reactions to the needles along her back, showing the muscles had relaxed. Her medication had been reduced and she had a new lease of life. We increased the interval between Kara's visits as long as she was happy and active. The spondylosis in her spine would never go away and could even worsen in the future, but after a three-month interval between treatments her mobility and weight were still good, so the decision was made to stop acupuncture. Her owners Joe and Carol know it is an option for the future, but I can't help but feel proud of them for achieving and maintaining Kara's ideal weight!

The key to weight loss for people and animals, when required, can be made simple by a change in routine. What that change should be can vary. It may be to stop ad-lib feeding, where food is left down twenty-four hours a day. This may be fine for cats, who seem better at self-regulation, but it's easy to overfeed a dog this way. If a dog is changed from ad lib to measured meals, once or twice a day, it gives much better control. It may be that leaving food down can make us feel better if our pet is left alone for a period of time, and it's possible that we mistake attention-seeking for food-seeking – there are lots of variables. While the cases I am sharing here are canine, many of the principles of feeding apply to cats too. With their different dietary requirements and tastes, I don't usually advocate the veggie option for them, although my vet friend Teresa, when reading an early draft of this book, told me that her cat steals peas – sometimes from her plate!

Springer Spaniel Tess was carrying some excess weight which wasn't helping her arthritic knees, but her owner Mac was struggling to feed her less. However one day she weighed in at the practice one-and-a-half kilos lighter than normal. When I asked what the difference was, Mac looked puzzled and said there had been no change. Until he realised that in the two months since I'd last seen Tess he had run out of dry food and had been feeding her tinned food only. That was what had made the difference. Dry food is condensed; it doesn't look much, but a small amount has a lot of calories.

I was hopeful that this would be the key to another dog's weight loss. Labradoodle Ness weighed in at forty kilograms and had no waist. Having started an acupuncture course to help with lameness, her weight record hadn't changed for three months. When we discussed it, Ness's owner said he was feeding her dry food, but realised that he had never had an overweight dog before and had always fed them wet food. He left that evening determined to buy some wet food. The result over time was excellent! Ness went on to lose around four kilos, approximately the equivalent of a dress size for a woman!

Regarding dry food? I was worried when, on holiday in Lanzarote, I watched some stray cats. They seemed to be content enough, were well fed, and no longer pestered visitors for scraps, but some of them were starting to fill out too much. A local charity was leaving dry food out for them, to help themselves to, and obviously some must have been doing so more than others. In some instances, dry food can be linked to the development of crystals or stones in the bladder in cats, and – at worst – can cause blockages. I tried not to think about what could happen if a cat developed cystitis in Lanzarote's hot, dry climate. But sometimes there are just too many 'what ifs' to worry about ...

As for Border Terrier Rhua, she lost ten per cent of her body weight simply because her owner June stopped feeding her treats when they were in the park. June hadn't realised how fattening the treats were and decided it was easier to cut them out completely during their walks, just making a bigger fuss of Rhua when she came back to her. Overall, Rhua had responded well to

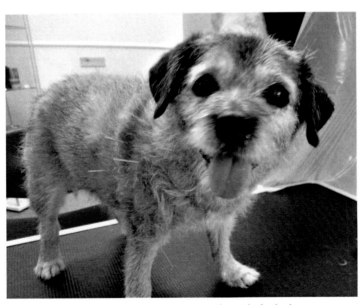

Rhua with needles in place to treat her right forelimb.

acupuncture for forelimb lameness, but she often hung back on her walks. It was only after the treats stopped that June realised Rhua had been very crafty. She had purposefully been hanging behind because she knew June would produce a treat to entice her to come. With no more treats, Rhua stopped lagging behind and instead began leading the way! At the ripe age of sixteen, Rhua is still going strong, albeit a little slower.

Rhua was one of four dogs under my care that came along to a talk I gave to vets and nurses on what acupuncture can do. One Labrador, Skye, had always been kept slim but Rhua, Pickles and Peanut had all lost between one and three kilograms. Passing round the equivalent weights in bags of food was met by gasps from the audience. It really hits home when you hold in your hands something equivalent to the weight loss, but I think it is best done after the weight loss has happened, in celebration, rather than before which is too daunting!

Despite the successes outlined above with vegetables, they are not the solution for every dog. Some simply don't like them. Fergus, a Standard Dachshund, will eat them, but his owner often finds them regurgitated on the floor in the morning. Fergus has been losing weight since his owner Frances started measuring out his daily food portion by portion, and any treats are taken from that – he does not get extras. In my view, portion sizes often have to be adjusted because the manufacturer's guidelines tend to recommend a bigger quantity than strictly necessary. Chocolate Lab Rolli lost four kilograms simply by his food portion being reduced from the recommended eighty to seventy grams. Labradors Maddie and Flynn, aged 11 and 12 (*opposite*), have come together for acupuncture for some years to help their mobility. Over this time they have lost a total of seven kilos each, since their owners George and Eleanor cut out treats. Maddie in particular has an insatiable appetite, as many Labradors do. Recently this has been attributed to a certain gene in their makeup, but it does not mean they actually need more calories!

The average weight of any given breed varies greatly, and the quantity of food needed also varies, influenced, for example, by the level of the animal's activity and whether it has been neutered, which can lower the metabolic rate. A vet friend in New Zealand reminisced about her father recently; he was more of a large-animal practitioner who worked in East Fife up to the 1980s, and used to say to the owners of overweight dogs, 'Give them a Smartie at the top of Largo Law a

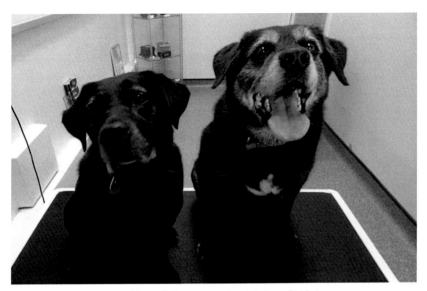

Maddie and Flynn – a total weight loss of 14 kg!

few times a week'. The dog was to get this single treat every time they walked up the three hundred-metre hill. And the owner would get a great view of the Firth of Forth!

When it comes to humans, the press tells us how obese our nation is nowadays. Around ten per cent of NHS funding in 2018 was spent on type 2 diabetes which is preventable through diet. It isn't just happening in the UK – increasing obesity, diabetes and heart disease are a world-wide problem linked to our more sedentary lifestyles and readily available high-calorie foods in developed and developing countries. The same happens when these 'foods' are introduced to indigenous populations. Our pet population merely follows the trend although, luckily for them, overconsumption of alcohol is not an issue! In his book *Doctor in the Wilderness* published in 1993, Perthshire GP Dr Walter Yellowlees described the unhealthy changes he observed in his patients in the 1950s and 60s following the introduction of white flour and sugar. He relates the case of two brothers, both farmers, who developed scurvy. Despite growing plenty of green vegetables, they deemed them to be cattle fodder and didn't eat any themselves. Dr Yellowlees was an advocate of growing your own food and avoiding damage to the soil by not over-farming and using fewer pesticides.

I think of how inspiring vet nurse Tricia is, having lost four stones over an eighteen-month period. She was motivated by her sore knees, which are a lot better as a result. My school friend Lindsay is now facing a dilemma, having hit the twenty-one-stone mark; he has been told by his doctor that his blood glucose levels and blood pressure are above normal and that weight loss is essential. He is starting to lose weight and hopefully can continue, like Tricia. Because Lindsay brought up the subject, I lent him my favourite local walking book which may mean that his Labradoodle Roxy will get some interesting walks to help reduce her waistline too! GP Liz recounts the tale of an American doctor who encouraged a patient to walk to a different pub at increasing distances away from home. The result was a decrease in both weight and alcohol consumption as more time was taken up by walking in the outdoors, rather than drinking and it was sustainable because he enjoyed his new way of life. The key is to find 'liveable' changes that can last and make a difference.

With all this talk of weight loss you might expect me to be some authority on the subject, with a sylph-like figure. However, by nature I am a human Labrador. I eat everything and leave nothing, and I can't bear waste! For some reason (probably several) I am very different from my brother. Ron is fair and slim and always has been, whereas I am dark and chunky and always have been, forever trying to slim or to stay slim. As a child I would eat everything in front of me, whereas Ron rebelled. There were so many things he wouldn't eat and any decisions on going out for a family meal or when we were on holiday revolved around what food would be acceptable to him. He lived on chips and ice cream on one of our two-week holidays. He would be taken to see the doctor every now and again because he was small and skinny, but Mum was always told that his diet was perfectly okay – comprising mostly peanuts, grapes, mince or corned beef with potatoes and baked beans. To this day he is still fussy and still doesn't eat eggs, but he is six-feet tall, fit and slim and feels that if he starts to put on any weight then the answer is simple – he eats less!

While I could go on about healthy eating for people and pets forever, it seems that finding a happy balance is the key between food and exercise. I was disturbed when I described how fussy one friend of mine is about eating 'healthy' food to my niece Diane. She often updates me on various matters 'some more obscure than others', and told me it sounded like she had orthorexia. "Ortho what?" I asked. Diane explained: it is a lesser-known eating disorder with a component of obsessive–compulsiveness in which the person is overly concerned and anxious about what is in their food, where it comes from, and how it has been prepared. With so much information available to us at the touch of a button, and conclusions that even the medical profession cannot agree on, is it so surprising that some of us overthink and develop this type of eating disorder?

With pets, concerns relate to whether a diet of raw food is better than processed. A while ago, after meeting an Australian vet who believed that processed food is detrimental, I looked into it further. I am old enough to remember seeing crumbly white dog faeces on the pavements at a time when many dogs were fed on bones and scraps from the butchers; this was before processed food and BSE put a stop to it. The white came from the undigested bony remnants. As Liz comments, they looked like miniature statues of poodles – and they didn't mess your shoes! But I also remember as a young graduate that bones could get trapped and cause untold damage. Bones can get stuck between teeth, across the roof of the mouth, and anywhere in the digestive tract. If they are sharp, they can cause perforations and sometimes irreparable damage. Attending a house visit on my first job, I had to remove spicules of bone by hand from a dog's bleeding bottom. Since those days, pet-food manufacturers have done a great deal of research developing complete foods for our domestic dogs and cats. Yet since graduating in 1983, obesity and dental disease have become far more common; in my opinion, this is linked to feeding more processed food.

When I returned to practice after some years out, I was aware of the debates about raw versus processed food. I had an open mind about raw food, however one of the first cases I saw was two cats recovering from a nasty *Salmonella* infection after being fed raw chicken. Just recently, one owner said she still wondered if a raw-food diet would be better for her dogs but admitted that she had picked up a *Campylobacter* infection in the past when she had started to use a raw preparation with her dogs. Nowadays there are many different raw-food preparations being used, but my PhD studies on bacteria and antibiotic resistance have made me more aware of the bacteria that can lurk in uncooked or improperly cooked meat, including *E. coli*

O157 and *Campylobacter*, as well as *Salmonella*, all of which can infect humans and cause serious illness. Multi-resistant bacteria have been isolated from raw dog food too, but the latest bacterial disease to cause concern, with an increasing number of reports in the veterinary news, is tuberculosis (TB) in cats (caused by the bacterium *Mycobacterium bovis)*, which was rarely reported previously. An investigation into a cluster of five cases of TB among indoor cats deduced that the only common denominator was the raw-meat diet they ate, implying that the *M. bovis* had been ingested in the beef from an infected cow.

An overactive thyroid gland (hyperthyroidism) is a common hormonal problem in cats, usually of undetermined cause (and in dogs, too, but it is rarer and more often linked to cancer). There are reports, however, that in some canine cases there is a link to feeding raw or canned dog food that contains the thyroid tissue of cows.

I mostly fed sachets of cat food to my own cat, who became hyperthyroidic when he was fifteen, but I think in general a mixture of dry and wet food for most dogs and cats is the happy medium. For all the reasons above, I have many reservations about feeding raw food. At the time of writing, Guinness has reached the age of at least nineteen, and still has a healthy appetite despite being almost toothless. He lost nearly a kilogram in weight and his lameness improved when we stopped giving him his portion of dry food. It may be that if he had not been fed on processed food he would still have all his teeth, but he once broke one of his canines when I tried experimenting with raw chicken.

Of course, many animals with access to plentiful food do not over-eat. I remember being incredulous as several boxed pizzas were laid out across the floor in the staff room when I was due to give a very informal lunchtime talk to a vet practice on the benefits of acupuncture. As the boxes were opened and the tantalising strong smells filled the room, I realised a black Labrador and a Spaniel were also loose in the room, so I was going to make a dash to lift the pizzas out of their way.

"No need," said one of the nurses. "Jake isn't interested in food and Dylan lives with vet Jenni and her family of three children and has been trained not to eat human food."

I was speechless! Jake was one of the slimmest Labs, but it was so unusual for that breed to be disinterested in food. He can't have been carrying the 'gorging' gene! Spaniel Dylan had been so well trained that he must have recognised that the smells, which were intoxicating to me, were not food for him!

For myself, I have learned that even when I exercise, if I consume too many calories I don't lose weight and even put it on. After completing my one-and-only Half Ironman triathlon two years ago, my 'resting-and-eating-what-I-like' period extended to three months and I put back on the stone I had lost. My five-kilometre park-run personal best time has latterly increased by five minutes and, while I hope to be fit for my annual hill-walking week in the north-west mountains of Scotland, which I love, I know there will be greater ease of movement and that the long days will be more enjoyable if I am carrying less weight in my 'rucksack'. You can guess what my New Year resolution is every year! I don't have an owner to ration me – the 'owner' is me!

— 14 —
Maintenance—Labradors, Retrievers (and the NHS)

Old dogs, like old shoes, are comfortable. They may be a bit out of shape and a little worn around the edges, but they fit well.

Bonnie Wilcox, author of *Old Dog, Old Friends*

Labradors are one of the most popular breeds of dog in the UK. For them, arthritis is the most common cause of debility affecting their quality of life, so it is no surprise that they are often acupuncture cases. Mac the chocolate Lab came for acupuncture for six years. He had multiple joints affected by arthritis and we had no idea how it quickly it would progress. When his eyesight began to deteriorate he underwent investigations to determine whether he was a candidate for cataract surgery to remove the milky white lenses that prevent light

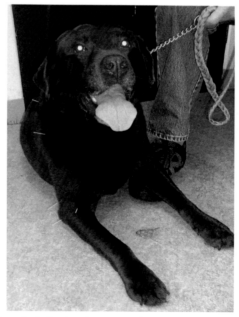

Mac who had cataract surgery – a long-term acupuncture patient completely unbothered by the needles.

from entering his eyes. It was a dilemma for his owners when deciding to put him through an operation because of his reducing mobility. However, when Mac was struggling to see his way in the dark, and even to find his food, the choice was made. Surgery it was. Mac never looked back, I am glad to say, and had the second eye operated on too. His restored sight restored his quality of life until he reached the age of fourteen and was finally unable to get up. His owners Dave and Carol, maintain he would never have got so far without acupuncture.

I still treat Cass, another chocolate Lab, not unlike Mac, who is nearing the age of fifteen and has several disfigured joints. At a recent visit I felt her head was wet.

"That's because she's been rolling on her back in the grass," owner Noel told me. We agreed that was a good measure of her quality of life. While she had a slow awkward gait she could still enjoy a roll.

Black Lab Rosie, also nearing fifteen, comes for acupuncture every six weeks or so, and has hydrotherapy in between sessions. She loves swimming, and the hydrotherapist is astounded at what she can manage at her age.

While some animals like Mac, Cass and Rosie, can get through a long life with no major incidents, there are others like Kola and Flora who have histories that astound their owners, and their vets and the nursing staff.

Kola

Owner Alison knew acupuncture was available in the practice, but when it was recommended for her yellow Lab, Kola, she had her doubts. Kola became nervous and scared and would shake when coming into the vets, so Alison and vet nurse Helaina, who knew Kola well, decided they should both be with her for her initial consultation.

Kola had good reason to be wary of the vets – she had been there so often. Some animals, like some people, seem luckier than others and only need routine procedures and vaccinations, but for others, ailments just keep on appearing and that was the way it was for Kola. She was unwell at her first visit at eight weeks old when she had only been in her new home for two days. The problems began with conjunctivitis, where her eyelids were swollen and weepy, and she was prescribed antibiotic eye cream. Then she became very dull and quiet and walked stiffly. She had a raised temperature and blood samples showed the possibility of infection and mild anaemia, so she was treated with antibiotics. But when swellings began to appear on her body something else was obviously the problem and an emergency appointment was arranged at Glasgow vet school. X-rays revealed changes in her bones due to inflammation. No bacteria were found in the skin lumps and a diagnosis of juvenile cellulitis was made, otherwise known as 'puppy strangles'. This is an uncommon but potentially serious disease of young pups in which there is a severe dermatitis. The treatment was high-dose steroids plus stomach-protective tablets and antibiotics. There is no known cause for strangles, but it may be caused by a problem with the immune system. Some breeds are more likely to succumb to it than others.

Kola responded to treatment well and got a good report at her check-up at the vet school one month later. However, just two weeks after that she let out a scream in the garden. She had fallen over and was holding up her left front leg. Unbelievably, a simple fall had resulted in a broken elbow. It is possible that the steroids had weakened her bones as she was showing signs of other side effects including a pot belly and thinning fur. She had needed the treatment for her strangles; however, sometimes side effects can't be avoided and can bring their own problems. Kola was referred again, this time to an orthopaedic specialist who confirmed the practice's findings. She had fractured the condyle (the part that sticks out) on the inside of her elbow joint. This presented a dilemma for Alison and Paul; they were due to go on holiday the next day and were thinking they would have to cancel. However, they were assured that for Kola an extended stay in hospital – for ten days instead of two – would mean it would be easy to keep Kola rested and thus aid her recovery. Surgery went well with three screws fixing the fracture in place although sometimes this type of fracture repair doesn't heal well and may increase the chance of osteoarthritis developing in future. It was an extra special homecoming for Alison and Paul to find Kola well on the mend.

Instead of vaccination at the usual two months of age, Kola was four months old before she was fit enough to have it. At her orthopaedic check, the screws were nicely in place and, although there were already some small early signs of arthritis, she was back to normal. But life was never uneventful for her. It seemed that every few months some ailment occurred. She had a false pregnancy before she could be spayed. It made her very out of sorts and put her off her food.

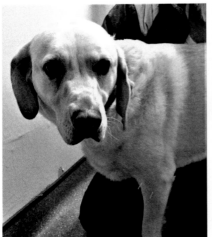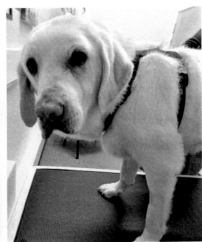

Kola having her elbow treated in 2011 (left) and on another visit in 2019 (right).

Numerous times she had treatment for other conditions – stitches for a cut pad or a dog bite; a torn claw; blood in her stools as she passed a stick she had chewed; allergic reactions to things unknown (once when her face swelled after she stuck her nose into piles of seaweed on a beach) – to name just a few.

Five years had passed since Kola's broken elbow when she started holding up the front leg on her left side. An x-ray showed more advanced changes typical of osteoarthritis in the elbow joint, as had been predicted. There were also some arthritic changes to the metacarpal joints of both her front feet (the small joints, equivalent to those in our hands). She had started a course of anti-inflammatories but although she improved, she was still limping. Due to her sensitive case history she was an ideal candidate for acupuncture.

Of course we had no idea how she would react to acupuncture, so Helaina cuddled her closely on the floor against the wall. However, our concerns were unfounded. Kola sat, then stood – quite the thing. I treated her thoracic spine and was able to circle her left elbow and hind leg points. She flinched a little at some points and was aware of the elbow ones, but stood quietly throughout, allowing me to treat LI4 at the web of her 'dew' claw – she was an ideal candidate! Afterwards, Alison said Kola had a mad session with her littermate brother, then limped again that night on her left foreleg. She'd also run after a

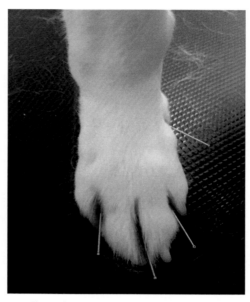

Needles in the Baxi points helped Kola's arthritic toes.

ball, then stopped and bolted into the house, possibly in response to pain. She recovered quickly from these incidents, however, and had been her usual grumpy self with the other dogs and growling, behaviours that had started some months before, also possibly due to pain.

By her fourth session Kola was quite happy coming into the practice. She had become much more relaxed on her visits and her tail wagged during the treatment. Kola would pull at her lead to come into my room and Helaina only needed to be there for reassurance the very first time. Kola was much better back at home, running around, no longer holding up her paw, with no obvious signs of pain, but sometimes she was very slow and occasionally grumpy with other dogs. I included some points on her head to see if that would help, and Alison was also trying out a pheromone diffuser at home. There were no sensitive areas at her elbow so reduction of her medication was planned. The intervals between acupuncture sessions increased and when Alison hadn't seen any limping after a four-hour walk, the interval was extended to six weeks. And once again, Kola would be pulling at her lead to come into my room!

But in 2014 she fractured a toe, on her right front leg. X-rays also showed severe osteoarthritis with newly laid-down bony growths, which explained why her front feet now spread out like a camel's. So I began treating her toes with acupuncture, which she did not seem to mind. Toe points can be very sensitive, as you can imagine! On discussing another dog with similarly affected paws some years ago, acupuncture vet Ann helpfully sent me a fax with a map of the feet showing the location of the Chinese Baxi points, located in the webs between the toes, which can be used on front or hind paws to help with conditions of the lower limbs. Sometimes I can't use them when I would like to – not every dog is accepting of them – and I have never tried with a cat!

Kola recovered well from her fractured toe and continuing acupuncture helped manage the arthritis, but the next year brought an even bigger challenge to her health.

On 1 July 2015 Alison and Paul noticed Kola had begun walking in a strange manner. When she was examined at the practice, she had a hypermetric gait. It looked like she was goose-stepping, and all four paws were knuckled over as if she didn't know where they were. Even if she had spondylosis at this point, such severe neurological changes wouldn't be expected. It was likely that she had a problem high up in the spinal cord, at the neck, so she was admitted to the practice for sedation, pain control and further investigation. The next day her condition was much worse. Moving her head was very painful for her and all four of her legs were knuckling under. A decision for referral was made.

She was admitted as an emergency case to the Glasgow vet school. By this time she was unable to walk as all four limbs were affected by some form of paralysis, worse on the left side. Under general anaesthesia, an MRI scan of the cervical spine revealed extensive material at vertebrae C5/7 in her neck, with distortion of the C6/7 joint and adjacent passageway for the spinal cord, causing pressure on the cord. This meant that Kola had two 'slipped discs' with bleeding and suspected malformation of the C6/7 joint. She needed emergency surgery.

The dorsal laminectomy operation meant that a large amount of disc material could be removed, which took the pressure off the spinal cord that was causing the paralysis. There was some concern about the amount of bleeding at the site; the forty-eight hours following surgery were critical. Six days later, Kola was able to go home, by which time she was walking well. A gradual improvement was anticipated, but Kola was under strict instructions to get full rest for four to six weeks

– which meant being confined to a small non-slip area, allowed out to toilet only, on a lead and harness, and not allowed to run, jump, play, or go up and down stairs. Alison and husband Paul had their work cut out!

When I eventually saw Kola again for acupuncture, she had made a good recovery from the surgery. If it weren't for the large shaved area and wound at her neck, I wouldn't have known anything had been amiss. She even jumped up onto the low table before we could stop her. She had been tiptoeing on her left foreleg, but that had completely resolved. I avoided her surgical site and repeated the usual acupuncture points for her left leg and toes.

Kola had been very lucky that such a serious and sudden-onset event did not result in permanent changes to the spinal cord. That was thanks to the prompt diagnosis and quick decision to operate. She has never looked back and, in December 2018, more than eight years since starting acupuncture, she still comes to me every seven to eight weeks – a great example of what acupuncture is capable of. Kola is also a great example of the benefits of modern surgical techniques that repaired her fractured leg and corrected a serious disc problem.

When Alison thinks of the tortuous way her five-year-old dog had plodded along, she never imagined in her wildest dreams that Kola would be so good at thirteen and a half. Had I heard her correctly when she said that Kola had been out for eighteen holes of golf four days in a row that week? Yes, I had! Other dog walkers who see Kola dashing along the beach are amazed when their estimate of how old she is has to be doubled. Alison has no doubt that the acupuncture contributes to her mobility, energy and general enjoyment of life!

Flora

Flora was a Flatcoat Retriever and was another ideal acupuncture candidate. Already x-rayed and referred by her vet Angus at Lomond Hills surgery, her elbows and knees were clear, but there was moderate to severe spondylosis of her spine that extended from the lumbar to the thoracic area, with some bony bridges between the vertebrae. Her spine was less flexible than it should be and she also had mild hip dysplasia, but the specialist orthopaedic vet who reviewed the x-rays was not convinced these changes were responsible for all her clinical signs. Her main symptoms were generalised stiffness and occasional lameness, so an MRI scan was needed to rule out narrowing of the

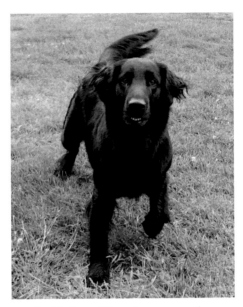

Kevin's photo of Flora at seven years of age.

spinal canal or disc problems, even though these scenarios were considered unlikely. She was not in severe pain or showing any nerve problems, but based on the x-rays and her clinical history, it was predicted that she would always have some niggling stiffness or discomfort and might be prone to flare-ups.

Flora's owner, Kevin, was doing as much as he could for his seven-year-old pet and in April 2014, when I met them, she was already on a special diet and supplement for her joints and was occasionally given the anti-inflammatory Previcox™. Kevin knew the breed very well – he had three of them – but he described Flora as 'always being a stiff dog' and 'limpy' from the age of one or two years. He had been advised to avoid high-impact exercise with her, especially twisting and turning movements, and had already stopped her jumping up into the car and playing ball. Despite all these precautions, her cycles of stiffness were becoming more frequent, and she often walked as if her legs were heavy. Kevin was concerned about the impact on her quality of life and was keen to avoid increasing medication.

At her first acupuncture treatment, Flora made an impressive entrance because of her large size and pure black fur. When I examined her, her ears were wet, and I asked Kevin why that was. Kevin explained that one of his other dogs liked to chew them – I don't think I would ever have guessed that reason! She was somewhat fidgety to begin with, wanting to keep moving round the room, so Kevin sat on a chair with her in the corner. Her spinal muscles were very tense and a strong twitch reaction bent one of the lumbar needles. Otherwise, she took it all in her stride. She was fine with acupuncture for her back and hips. As the number of sessions mounted up, she was quite self-contained, neither up nor down, and often just relaxed, lying on her side.

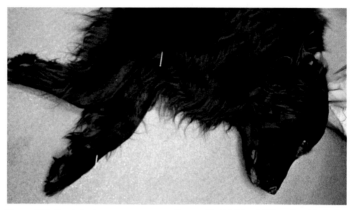

Flora chilled out during acupuncture – the needles highly visible in her black fur.

Because Kevin described the stiffness coming in cycles, I expected it to take a couple of months before we knew whether acupuncture was helping her, but in fact there were positive indications early on. Flora was stretching out more when she lay on the floor, and was enjoying her normal walks. She'd even chased a deer with one of the younger dogs – something she hadn't done for a while. Using his own scoring system, Kevin rated her at nine out of ten and felt overall he was managing her condition well, just using the Previcox™ when she overdid things.

Flora continued to have acupuncture every four weeks or so for two years, but as she got older daily medication was needed to maintain a more constant concentration of the drug in her blood stream, to provide more even anti-inflammatory control. Her condition was pretty stable until January 2017, when she became unwell and had a vaginal discharge that extended beyond the usual length of her season. Vet Angus diagnosed pyometra, a very common but life-threatening condition in which there are changes to the uterus. Surgery was carried out to remove it. Angus commented about the extent of Flora's spondylosis that he saw during the operation – he'd never seen anything like it – he could feel the bone spurs from her lumbar vertebrae protruding into her abdomen. The extent of this can be seen marked by the arrows on the x-ray below.

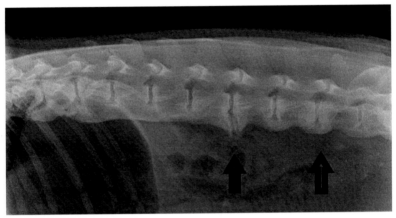

Flora's extensive spondylosis with bridges of bone between the vertebrae.
Courtesy of Lomond Hills Veterinary Clinic.

Kevin was concerned about how she would cope with the operation, given her age and condition, but at her next acupuncture session, I wouldn't have known she had undergone major surgery if it hadn't been for her shaved belly and healed wound. Flora appeared to be back to her usual self. Little did we know what lay ahead, though.

Within a couple of months she began to have an occasional cough and slightly heavy breathing. These signs are typical of the start of laryngeal paralysis, where parts of the larynx or windpipe collapse inward and narrow the passage for breathing. It is potentially life-threatening if it progresses but it can remain stable for some time. Flora's medication had to be changed to steroids and a different type of painkiller to avoid interaction with the Previcox™ she was on, and I also added acupuncture points that help with breathing.

Meanwhile, two lumps were found in her mammary glands following biopsies in May 2017. They revealed cancer, so she underwent another operation to remove them. By this time she was even stiffer and taking even more medication. No measurable difference was noted when we tried using laser acupuncture instead of needles; we had to accept that Flora had plateaued after the surgery.

The following June, in 2018, there were yet more concerns. Her mobility had deteriorated and she was drinking and urinating more. Her anti-inflammatories were stopped because of the effect they might be having on her kidney function. Angus found on an ultra-sound scan that one of Flora's kidneys had shrunk, and diabetes insipidus was diagnosed after further tests. This meant her kidneys had lost the ability to concentrate urine, hence her need to urinate more. Fortunately the diabetes responded to treatment, although having a urinary tract infection at the same time didn't help. Yet Flora just kept going! Despite the many ups and downs, Kevin always felt that Flora picked up after acupuncture. I could only marvel at her stoicism.

By the October, Flora's respiratory noises were increasing – the laryngeal paralysis was progressing. An inhaler had been tried without success, so we discussed referral and the possibility of surgery if she deteriorated, but Flora had already been through so much that Angus preferred to try another medication, a bronchodilator, to help open up the airways. By November, Flora seemed perkier. Her breathing had settled and her mobility was stable. When she came for acupuncture in December, she was managing reasonably well on low-dose steroids. She had only occasional breathless episodes and the steroids seemed to be helping her mobility too. After a lot of discussion, because her laryngeal condition was potentially life-threatening, Kevin decided Flora should go for further investigations so we discussed the options again. Angus had arranged for her to be assessed the following day for laryngeal surgery by a visiting specialist. Then Kevin mentioned that one of her eyes didn't look quite right.

I had watched Flora's movements as she came in, then greeted her and prepared for her acupuncture, but I hadn't noticed anything amiss with her eye. From a distance her face was just all black, but when I took a close-up look, I saw that her left eye was different from the right. It wasn't conjunctivitis, which is inflammation of the eyelids and quite common; it seemed that her eyeball was larger than it should be. Anything that causes the eyeball to increase in size is a worry. As I compared her eyes, I applied a little pressure to the top of the upper eyelid; the tension in the eyeball didn't feel abnormal, which suggested that the problem wasn't glaucoma, where the eyeball swells because of a build-up of fluid inside, and Flora didn't pull back as if she was in pain.

Still, the left eyeball was definitely protruding. The 'white of the eye' area was more visible than on the right eye – something was pushing the eye forward. My heart sank. There had to be something behind the eye, occupying space. The most likely cause was some sort of growth, but I was hesitant to mention that because there are other possibilities. I alerted Angus's practice that Flora would need to be seen before going to the laryngeal assessment the following day. Despite everything she had been through, this was yet another challenge.

So Flora went back to Angus again. Her laryngeal assessment was cancelled and her head was scanned instead. She had a mass behind her left eye. The next time I saw her, her mobility was the same but she was making more respiratory noise, and her eye was protruding more. It was also a little ulcerated. While we were all getting boxed into corners about the next best course of action, Flora was lively and happy in herself. She had none of the angst that Kevin had when they went back to see Angus again.

At Flora's next acupuncture treatment her bouts of heavy raspy breathing were alarming. Even though she was making a quick recovery from these bouts, it indicated that her airway was narrowing yet further. It felt ironic this was all going on while we were still waiting for the results of the biopsy taken from behind her eye. At this treatment session, I included needles around the troubled eye in an effort to reduce swelling in the cheek below. That swelling indicated the tumour was getting bigger, whereby the increasing pressure was causing some fluid retention in the skin.

The biopsy revealed a carcinosarcoma, a malignant mixed tumour, a kind of tumour that has more than one cell type and is usually aggressive. Angus operated to remove Flora's left eye along with some of the tumour tissue, however it had been impossible to remove all of it – it was such a tangled web.

Two weeks after the surgery Flora strode confidently into the consulting room as if nothing had happened. I was nothing short of amazed! She had another patch of shaved skin and a neat wound where her eye had been, but had been 'on the go' as usual. I was still concerned by her breathing – it was much louder by the end of that session. The following month Kevin told me he was pleased about how well she was coping with it all, but we knew she was on borrowed time. There seemed to be a little more swelling on her left cheek, but otherwise Flora was still enjoying life and eating well.

On her many visits over the years, I had sometimes wondered during one of her health challenges if it was the last time I would see her. But my notes include comments like 'happy in self', 'minimal needling reactions', 'relatively full of beans' and so on. Then in March 2019 I received an email from Kevin. My heart sank. She had had a breathing crisis.

> Hi Jane
>
> I'm afraid that we had to euthanise Flora last night. Angus was as fantastic as he always is and Flora had a happy, gentle death (as indeed we would wish for us all).
>
> What can I say? Thank you, thank you, thank you.
>
> In hindsight, Flora had obvious symptoms of her spinal condition from about the age of two. At the age of six her spondylosis was diagnosed as severe. Between you, me and Angus, we took a dog with really pretty bad spinal issues and gave her a pretty normal and active life all the way through to age twelve. I think that we have all (including obviously Flora) done magnificently well.
>
> Words cannot express how grateful I am to you. I hope that it goes without saying that it has been a pleasure to get to know you over the last few years.
>
> Kind regards,
>
> Kevin

I was going to miss Flora – and Kevin.

More about Kola

I thought I had finished Kola's story in December 2018 when I wrote about her being out on the golf course, and that would have been a nice place to stop – but it was not to be. Six weeks after that happened, at her routine weigh-in before acupuncture, she had lost weight. Her owner Alison was surprised and didn't know why. Unintentional weight loss, especially in an older dog whose activity has not increased, always rings alarm bells for a vet because there is often a sinister reason.

On questioning Alison, she described some unusual behaviour. Kola would bark halfway through eating her meal and then, instead of eating it all in one go as usual, she would leave it, then go back to it after her bowl had been moved. She was also drinking more and was a bit unsteady on her legs at times. On feeling her abdomen, around the bladder area, something didn't feel quite right to me, so blood tests were arranged.

She had a high calcium blood level, indicative of a cancer somewhere. A scan revealed enlarged lymph nodes in her abdomen, then rectal examination revealed a large mass where an anal gland should be. She was quickly referred to the Dick vet school. The mass was cancerous, and enlarged lymph nodes near the spine, lung and kidney were confirmed – indicating metastases. The cancer had spread and it was aggressive.

The Dick vets explained the options in detail to Alison and Paul. If treated palliatively – meaning treating only the symptoms – Kola may not respond to the treatment for the high calcium level in her blood which was affecting her whole well-being and she could become unable to defecate as the anal mass enlarged. After a lot of soul-searching by Alison and Paul, Kola embarked on cancer treatment at the age of thirteen.

First her blood calcium level had to be stabilised, then two operations followed, the first to remove the anal gland mass – the source of the cancer – and the second to remove some lymphatic tissue. This was in March 2019. She made a good recovery, astounding the vets and nurses at the vet school. Kola was a star patient and was home again in no time, with her usual meloxicam and also gabapentin for her arthritic pain.

Kola subsequently started a long-term chemotherapy regimen with palladium, supportive medications and regular visits and blood tests at the Dick to monitor how she was coping. A course of radiotherapy was included, whereby radiation specifically targets the area of cancer. Kola had the most dedicated of owners and received the latest in medical care from the oncology team at the vet school; they described her in one report as 'a lovely dog and very brave for her investigations'. Kola just took everything in her stride and coped amazingly well. The cancer was being kept at bay.

Alison made sure we kept her acupuncture going. I noticed Kola's coat change colour, become paler, with a bald area over her rump where the skin was redder, and darker colouring around her nose – all side effects from her treatment. Not being involved in Kola's cancer treatment, it was difficult for me to comprehend what she had been and was going through; she had lost some weight but was just the same dog! We decided to keep on with the acupuncture to help her mobility, boost her immune system and help with pain control alongside all the medication she was on. With some strong twitch responses and awareness of the Baxi points in her paws, she continued to show a good response to acupuncture – there was nothing to lose.

Then, in the July, Kola became very lame on her left hind leg. She had ruptured the anterior cruciate ligament in her knee. Surgery is often needed when this happens because the joint becomes unstable; however, the vets at the Dick were reluctant to go down that route because of her ongoing chemotherapy treatment. The only option for her was strict rest, continuing pain medication and more frequent acupuncture. This we did, and I was astounded when Kola's lameness improved remarkably, within just a few weeks, and there was no need for her to have surgery!

However, this was only a lull in Kola's story. In August of that year there was a crisis. One evening Kola was taken to the veterinary emergency service. She was trying to vomit and her stomach was bloated. These are signs of gastric torsion (a twisted stomach), which is another life-threatening condition that requires major surgery and can often have complications. The vet listened as Alison recounted Kola's history and was leaning towards the option of putting her to sleep. However, Alison wasn't convinced it was Kola's time yet. And when Kola lifted up her head to look at her from the examination table, she took it as a sign to give her one last chance.

I certainly had my doubts when I saw Kola in the recovery ward the day after her surgery. She was lying flat out, panting heavily. But yet again, she made a remarkable recovery and was soon back for more acupuncture. Sometime later, a new 'growth' appeared, near one of her toes. I treated it by circling the dragon. Luckily it wasn't a cancer and it responded well and soon healed.

In February 2020, Kola was still being monitored by the Dick vets, and was still happy to come for acupuncture, constantly astounding everyone who knew about her medical history. Alison kept well, too. She had been under the care of the cardiology department at the local hospital when Kola was receiving her cancer treatment, where she had her pacemaker battery replaced surgically to keep her heart beating regularly. She had been diagnosed with a serious heart condition when Kola was only a year old. If the pacemaker hadn't worked, she would have needed a heart transplant. Luckily, the pacemaker did work, and her recovery from the operation had astounded her consultants as much as Kola's had astounded us. Alison told me that having Kola around had made a huge difference to her own wellbeing – she just had to keep going and be well enough to take Kola out for walks! I am full of admiration for two such resilient and positive characters.

Without having matching cases to compare with Flora and Kola (one that received acupuncture and the other not), it cannot be said categorically that the acupuncture had contributed to their good quality of life and longevity. Yet, after more than twenty years' experience of acupuncture, and witnessing and hearing the responses of numerous two and four-legged friends, I am sure that it does.

Tricia, the owner of Golden Retriever Archie, says she can't believe that at fourteen years old he isn't on any medication. Three years ago he seemed to be slowing up a little and taking longer to get up and down from a lying position, but he responded well to a course of acupuncture with top-ups every six to eight weeks.

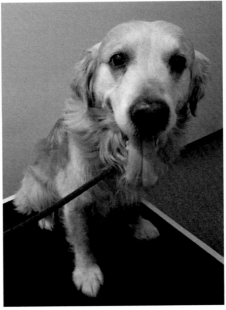

Archie at the age of fourteen.

Marge and Sylvia—more human patients

Much to her regret and annoyance, GP Liz had to stop offering acupuncture on the NHS due to lack of funding and time. While she had stopped taking on new patients, she had referred a few that she was already treating to me. So in 2005, I met Marge and Sylvia – I am still treating them, fifteen years later! They both have something to say about the human perspective. Here are their stories …

Marge was already a fan of acupuncture when she and her daughter Sylvia started coming to me for treatment. Marge recounts how, a long time ago, her very down-to-earth friend Isa described the pain of her frozen shoulder as being worse than any of the six births she had gone through, and that acupuncture worked wonders for her. What also impressed Marge was watching a TV programme about acupuncture in which a crippled horse miraculously ran around its field after its treatment. "There can't be any placebo effect on a horse," she stated forcefully.

Marge's first experience of acupuncture was over thirty years ago. Dr Eva Pitt at her local hospital treated her when she was diagnosed with ME (the chronically fatiguing and painful condition that has no known cause or cure). Acupuncture made her feel very much better. Since then her list of health issues has grown but her main problem is pain and stiffness, especially in her neck and lower back, and she has a tendency towards sciatic pain. Marge has always preferred laser acupuncture because she knew she couldn't cope with any potential discomfort caused by massage or needling. When she comes for treatment, I just follow her instructions as to what area is sorest and where to target! However, once there was a successful side issue. Marge told me about an irritating, unsightly patch of dermatitis on her hand, at the web between the first and second fingers of her right hand, about a centimetre in diameter. Sometimes it got a bit better but it never went away. She'd had it for decades and just assumed it was going to be there for life. I was telling her about some success I'd had with circling the dragon on scars and skin lumps when I began to realise there was nothing to lose in treating her hand. And she was keen! After circling several times around the edge with small needles, slowly but surely the scabbed area dried up and disappeared. That was a few years ago now and there is still no trace of it.

Back pain and stiffness had also plagued Marge's daughter Sylvia, ever since she'd had her second child over thirty years previously! She'd been unable to work for eighteen months afterwards and her back

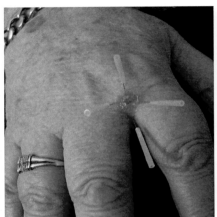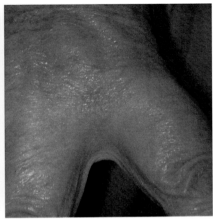

Marge's skin lesion which disappeared after acupuncture.

was still so stiff in the mornings that she couldn't bend down to put her clothes or footwear on. On occasion she'd had to ask a neighbour to help. Acupuncture made all the difference for her, and like her mum she prefers the laser option.

"Mind and say about my elbows," Sylvia piped up one day as she lay on the treatment table. She had a form of tennis elbow that I suspected was work-related; she worked in a biscuit factory lifting boxes repetitively. The pain woke her at night and it would take an hour or so until she could straighten her elbows out and the pain eased, before she could get back to sleep. If not for acupuncture, she says she could not have continued working.

GP Liz reports that she sees less of Marge and Sylvia nowadays, now they have regular laser acupuncture; they often used to consult with her about pain control. With an ageing population and the occurrence of more and more chronic conditions, it would make sense if acupuncture – in some form – was more readily available. Both humans and our domestic pets can benefit.

— 15 —

Keeping an open mind

In times of joy, all of us wished we possessed a tail we could wag.

W.H. Auden (poet, author and playwright)

Of course, some cases are more straightforward, especially when it comes to the use of acupuncture in pain management. Those of Paolo and Dawn were more of a challenge. Jarlath was approaching early retirement from his role in veterinary practice, unfortunately forced upon him by ill-health, at the age of fifty-three. I had been thanking him for his support of the acupuncture clinic as we reminisced about Oz and some of my other cases. He commented that one of the most important things he had learned during his career was to have an open mind. This has been a constant thread throughout these acupuncture stories, but the following cases are more recent and they remind me of the constant battle to keep an open mind and fend off my internal naysayer. The following story of Paolo and Dawn, followed by Petra and Craig's in Chapter 16, show where having an open mind can lead.

Paolo's pain and paralysis

One evening at the end of September 2017, Paolo, a French Bulldog who wasn't yet six years old, suddenly started crying and yelping every time he moved. He was miserable. Even food wouldn't tempt him to walk and he was being hand-fed. Paolo was taken to his vet the following day. On examination his tummy was relaxed, which ruled out an abdominal cause, but he screamed when he wriggled his body to escape from having his rectal temperature taken. He soon settled down and no pain was found when his neck was moved or pressure was applied along his back. It was all a bit confusing.

He was admitted into the clinic for further assessment and strong pain relief. It wasn't clear what was causing him so much pain, but it was suspected that he'd had too much 'rough and tumble' with the other dog he lived with and had injured himself. A spinal injury was the prime suspect, but other causes couldn't be ruled out. Only time would tell.

Later that day he seemed comfortable and was walking well so he was sent back home with instructions for strict rest. At his follow-up the next day, he was very much better. Although he was still hunched and moving stiffly, he wasn't screaming and even allowed his temperature to be checked. His temperature was normal, which ruled out infection, so more strict rest and continued pain relief were prescribed. He was still being offered food by hand so he didn't have to bend down, and was eating and toileting as usual.

Five days later Paolo's owners, Jackie and Alan, were worried because he was still having spasms of pain. He could walk for ten minutes on the lead without yelping, but then he wanted to go home. Stronger pain control was prescribed and ten days later, at his next check-up, he was back to normal.

Then two months later he had another scrap with the other family dog. This time the trauma was more obvious, with bruising and scrapes around his face, a puffy red eye and a sore back. Paolo was back at his vet's again, and more pain medication and rest was advised. Two weeks later he hadn't improved. He was still very sore and struggling to move. The vet noted some alarming new signs: he was reluctant to turn his head to the right, and was holding up his left front paw. The new concern was that he might have a disc problem. Another ten days later he had deteriorated, despite being kept in a cage at home to restrict his movements. He was given a higher dose of gabapentin for possible nerve pain, and Pardale™ (paracetamol and codeine) tablets. Paolo's neck was very sore, his head was constantly tipped to the left, putting a disc problem high on the list of possible diagnoses.

Two days later he was admitted for a general anaesthetic so that x-rays could be taken of his neck and thoracic spine. There was some difficulty interpreting them, though, because French Bulldogs do not have normal-shaped vertebrae; it is one of the drawbacks of their in-breeding, making them vulnerable to spinal conditions and injuries. While it was good that there were no signs of calcified discs or compression of the spinal cord, referral to a university hospital was the next step, to see a neurologist – in the first instance – and then to be assessed for surgery. However, Paolo's owners were reluctant to put him through too much.

At the end of February 2018, five months later, I took a call from Alan. He and Jackie were in a bit of a quandary as to what was best for Paolo. Overall, he seemed to be improving but occasionally he was racked with pain and had more bouts of screaming. Paolo was actually their son's dog, and had lived at the son's own home, but because the other dog could be aggressive – and was considered to be the cause of Paolo's injuries – they adopted Paolo in December to avoid putting him at more risk. He was leading the quietest of lives, and was still being hand-fed and cage-rested. At this stage, the only options were for further investigations and possible surgery. Jackie and Alan had to face the awful truth that, because of Paolo's pain and difficulty in walking, he may be better off put to sleep.

When I first met Paolo, Alan carried him into the practice. His black and white body looked small and vulnerable as he shrank into his owner's arms. In the previous six weeks or so he had been the best he had ever been, but hadn't fared well during the half-hour car journey, becoming anxious and unsettled. I was seeing him at his worst. My heart went out to him. When placed on the floor, he didn't want to move; his short neck was extended and rigid. When he did move it was only hesitantly; he dragged his left front leg which scuffed on the floor. This was a sure sign that there was nerve damage, most likely due to compression by a disc.

I hadn't seen an animal in so much pain for years. In fact, it was my human friend Sheryll, in New Zealand, that I'd last seen suffering that much, when she could hardly bear to move. Two of us had helped her along her hallway at home to the toilet, because even that simple task caused her a great deal of pain. She was told her back pain was muscular and to give it time, alongside pain medication. However, just a few weeks later she bent down to pick up some shopping and collapsed. She lost the use of her legs and bladder, which is an emergency arising from significant compression of the lower spinal cord, with the potential for permanent damage. Sheryll was taken to her local hospital and then transferred by air ambulance to a specialist unit in Wellington. Time was of the essence, and by road the journey would have taken two hours. During an emergency operation several discs were removed from her spine and luckily, although it took some time, she made a complete recovery. Even when someone can describe their pain, it isn't always obvious what the cause is. A 'wait and see' approach is often the only option until some critical sign appears.

Paolo's signs varied in severity, but he wasn't leading a normal life for a dog. Even if surgery was considered appropriate for him, which might cost thousands of pounds, there was no guarantee that he

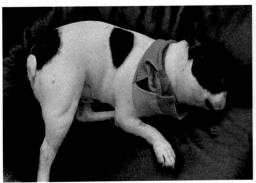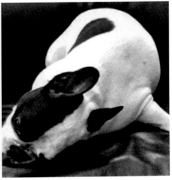

Photos taken at home by Jackie and Alan – Paolo's unusual posture.

would be restored to full fitness. In desperation, Jackie had found my details via the internet and Alan then called to ask if Paolo could have acupuncture – as a last resort – as he was showing little improvement with rest and pain relief. Paolo's regular vet felt there was nothing to lose if he had acupuncture alongside his current medication, so she referred him to me. She believed it would do no harm, but was sceptical about it helping his extreme pain. Based on his history, so was I. *Keep an open mind*, I told myself.

Paolo had received the best of available drugs at the time, including tramadol and steroids and gabapentin with diazepam for particularly severe spasms. They had helped to some extent but it felt to me that things could still get worse. What if the tight muscles close to his vertebrae and discs in his neck were actually stopping a disc from popping out completely, which I might loosen with acupuncture? That would be disastrous. So I decided to treat points away from his neck first. His owners felt it was worth trying, so Paolo was lifted onto the table. I explained that I couldn't make any promises because his was an extreme case and that if he got any worse after acupuncture then he would have to be referred – or a decision would be needed to let him go.

I wondered whether some of Paolo's problems were due to his breeding and reflected on our responsibility for introducing unhealthy traits into breeds – such as deformed vertebrae and short noses – just because they look cute. There is a specialist surgical unit at Cambridge vet school that deals purely with short-nosed dog breeds that have respiratory problems caused by narrowed airways and overly long soft palates.

Feeling reluctant to treat Paolo, because he had not had an MRI scan and I wasn't sure what I was dealing with, I held out little hope. Nonetheless, I agreed to treat him once. If he got worse, he would be referred, but if not we would give him a course of four treatments.

French Bulldogs have short thick necks. Paolo's felt like concrete. He twitched as if electric shocks were going through his head and neck. I began using very superficial acupuncture points, just through his skin and a little muscle, nearer to his tail than his head, and worked my way along his back, finishing with two needles in his head. By the end of the session we were amazed to see that he visibly relaxed and the twitchy spasms lessened. Apparently he slept all the way home in the car. That was the first day of his first acupuncture treatment, in March 2018.

When I next saw him, ten days later, his owners told me he had been brighter and more active, with no spasms of pain or yelping. He had walked along the corridor, his left fore-paw still knuckling and his head still tilting, but at least he was taking an interest in his surroundings and even lowered his head to sniff things. I breathed a sigh of relief. It was absolutely worth continuing his treatment, even though we didn't know whether it was just a good week or whether the acupuncture had already had an effect. I still felt uncomfortable going ahead without an MRI or diagnosis, but these things are not always possible. So we proceeded with the second treatment and I was delighted that his muscles seemed more relaxed. I did more points, which Paolo accepted, and included his left front leg, adding Chinese Baxi points at the webs of his toes. As you can imagine, animals and people are usually very sensitive having needles inserted between their toes, but Paolo wasn't bothered at all. It was as if he didn't feel them; unfortunately this was not a good sign because it indicated a lack of sensation in his foot.

Yet Paolo just kept improving. His medication was reduced and on the seventeenth day after his first treatment, he came for his third. He was more playful and had started barking again. He was getting cockier! He had been back to his own practice, too, where the vets and nurses were amazed by his improvement – as were Jackie and Alan. He corrected his left foreleg when it was put in a knuckling position, which meant he knew exactly where his paw was. He could look upwards, and he even took a treat from me. I felt confident enough to massage his neck and found the muscles were more relaxed and I was now able to insert two needles into this area. He had put on some weight during his convalescence but now, with less food and more exercise, his weight was steadily dropping again, and had gone below 15.3 kilos. He was transitioning away from being a patient, and Jackie and Alan were more and more confident about what they could let him do.

About three weeks later, Paolo had his fourth acupuncture session. He sprinted up the stairs into the surgery – so happy to come for acupuncture! He was now eating from a bowl with gusto, not tentatively by hand. There was less scuffing of his left leg, his head was less tilted and overall he was more stable. He could cock his leg again, without falling over. I was pleased by how relaxed he was during his treatment and the way he lay down soon after it began, and to see that he felt one of the needles when I inserted it near a toe.

By the end of May, about ten weeks after his first session, and five treatments later, he was off all medication. He was running around and springing onto the couch at home 'like a lamb', and onto the low table in the consulting room. His left front leg was completely normal and he didn't fall to one side when he shook himself. During his sixth treatment he yawned as he lay on his side with the needles in place, only showing awareness at some lumbar and knee points. This time, he pulled his leg away when I began to treat his foot, so I decided it wasn't needed – his sensation had been restored! As he sat on the floor afterwards, he looked up at me with a quizzical face, hoping for a treat. Apparently he had no neck pain either. I didn't see him for another month.

On day 111 after his first treatment, he was back for his seventh. Jackie and Alan described him as being back to normal, full of beans and running and jumping normally. He had just a little head tilt when he sneezed, but showed no unsteadiness after. Now weighing 14 kilos, he was slimmer; a weight of 13.5 kilos was the goal and he was nearly there. On repeating his needling he quickly settled and was nicely sleepy by the end of the session. I realised that this was it – the end of his treatment – but before I signed him off, I asked if I could see him again two months later. I wanted to be sure that everything was okay and not tempt fate!

By September 2018, Paolo's owners said he was 'fantastic'. He was at an ideal weight of 13.3 kilos, having lost exactly two – 13% of his body weight – since I'd first seen him. I did a last acupuncture treatment. He reacted a little to a needle in the left side of his back, which may have been because he still had a head tilt, however his neck was completely relaxed. We talked about the fact that his head tilt, which was likely to be permanent, was hardly noticeable and clearly not bothering him. The last report from Jackie and Alan was that Paolo is running full speed on the beach at the West Sands in St Andrews. He is back to being Paolo. Jackie and Alan know that the weight loss helps maintain his fitness but they put his near-complete recovery down to acupuncture.

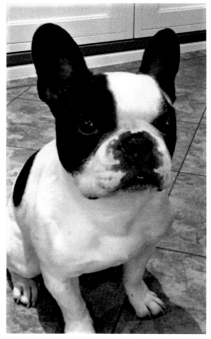

A recovered Paolo!

It is likely that the nerve damage to Paolo's leg was caused by compression from the tight injured muscles of his neck. This was released by acupuncture and healing was promoted. While I'm sorry that I don't see Paolo anymore, he has been one of my most rewarding cases and I hope not to see him back at the surgery any day soon!

Dawn and hyposmia

Here are some more definitions for you. 'Hyposmia' refers to a partial loss of the sense of smell. 'Anosmia' is the absence of sense of smell. And 'dysosmia' relates to a change in smell. 'Phantosmia' is smelling strange smells. When I first saw the word 'anosmia' written down, in an email from Jarlath, I nearly turned to my medical dictionary, but I was able to work out what it meant from other details he gave me. The email was quite out of the blue and a pleasant surprise. He had retired by then, and I had seen him only briefly since he'd left the practice some months before. Early retirement isn't much fun when the reason is the onset of Parkinson's disease. He was having a stressful time of it, having given up veterinary medicine and his long commitment to the practice. I thought he might be coming to me for a massage or some acupuncture, because we'd talked previously about how it might help with some of his shoulder tension – and I'd given him a gift voucher (for encouragement) when he left.

We'd also chatted about other people I knew with Parkinson's, including one of my veterinary clients, Rosie, who received her diagnosis shortly after retirement. Like Jarlath, she had put a lot of her symptoms – the unusual levels of fatigue and occasional muscular twinges – down to work stress. Rosie had seen her dogs, Blue and Skye, benefit from acupuncture, so she was keen to try it for herself. She found that the acupuncture pain and calf points I used, along with calf massage, helped to keep her cramps at bay. She kept fit by walking her dogs and going to regular Pilates classes, so her consultant had told her just to keep doing what she was doing. Unfortunately, there was nothing I could do to reduce the tremor in her hands.

My cousin Drew also had Parkinson's diagnosed when he lived in Cornwall, and was then medically retired from his driving job. He coped fine with just gentle massage – and literally shook with fear at the thought of needles! Acupuncture is not for everyone, of course, and he relies on golf and cycling as his tonics!

But Jarlath's email was not about treatment for himself or about any animal cases. He was hoping to help his wife.

Do you have any experience in treating people with anosmia with acupuncture? My wife Dawn has partially lost her sense of smell and taste for the last 18 months or so, probably post viral infection. Conventional treatment and investigations have been unsuccessful. I have read of some success in cases treated by acupuncture.

Regards
Jarlath

This was a new type of request. I knew acupuncture can be used for many, many different ailments – but being unable to smell? I replied to tell him I had no experience of anosmia but would find out which points to use and that it would be worth a try. The important facts to me were that Dawn was a nurse who had been through the NHS system and had no more options to explore. The prospect of acupuncture providing a solution gave me a 'pot of gold at the end of the rainbow' kind of feeling. And it gave me confidence that it was totally appropriate to try acupuncture for Dawn, knowing that Jarlath had seen for himself what acupuncture could do for animals.

I found some papers online, checked my textbooks and asked my GP acupuncture friend, Liz, if she knew anything about treating anosmia. "Oh, yes," she said and pointed to her face and head. "I've read about these points".

She hadn't been able to continue giving acupuncture within the NHS because of limitations in her available appointments, and funding, and the 'evidence for acupuncture' debates, but she had kept up her interest and was always a mine of information. The following Saturday I happened to be attending an acupuncture meeting in Uddingston, which was run by Susie, a retired NHS midwife and experienced acupuncturist who ran her own clinic. She had treated a patient who had lost her sense of smell towards the end of a cold, and acupuncture had certainly seemed to help her. I also found a case report in the *Acupuncture in Medicine* journal, which described the success of treating someone with anosmia. Armed with my research, I had made a note of the combination of points I would use. First I had to go through Dawn's history.

She had a minor cold, she said, not sinusitis (although I thought it sounded like it), and that was not normal for her. Since May of that year (about the same time of Jarlath's diagnosis) she had lost her sense of smell following a heavy viral cold. She had no history of head trauma or infection other than the cold, and she wasn't taking any medication that might cause loss of smell as a side effect. Her condition was classed as 'post-viral olfactory dysfunction' – PVOD for short. For three months she had been using a steroid nasal spray. She described how her sense of smell had changed: often smells were unusual or putrid and her sense of taste was also greatly reduced. Her ENT consultant had said everything was clear when a scope was passed along her nasal tubes – no nasal polyps. And an MRI scan of her brain was clear, meaning the possibility of a tumour in the olfactory (smell) lobes of her brain could be ruled out. There was some thickening of the tissue in one of her sinuses, so she had undergone tissue removal under general anaesthetic in case the thickened membranes would cause problems in the future. The procedure couldn't help her smell normally again. Then it was recommended that she contact Fifth Sense, a UK charity that provides support and advice to people suffering from smell and taste-related disorders. They advised trying to retrain her sense of smell by regularly sniffing clove, rose, eucalyptus and lemon oils.

Dawn felt despondent, knowing there were no other treatment options. She was smelling the oils, but could only faintly detect the eucalyptus and lemon; even though she knew what they were, she couldn't smell the rose or cloves. Because she could smell some things, she was labelled as having hyposmia rather than anosmia. So, despite having never had acupuncture before, she was more than happy to give it a go.

Dawn lay back on the couch in my room and kept perfectly still as I inserted the small needles, two points on either side of her nose (Large Intestine 20, or LI20). These are actually called the 'welcome fragrance' points in traditional Chinese acupuncture, and it felt good to use them. The other points on her face were situated mostly along the midline and they extended up into her scalp. Dawn seemed perfectly relaxed but I know about the giant leap of faith involved in coming for a totally different type of treatment. I was delighted when, a few days later, this email arrived.

> *Thought I'd drop you a wee update.*
>
> *Following my treatment session on Wednesday there's been a noticeable improvement! I was definitely able to smell the bakery in the supermarket – I felt quite emotional and was sure I looked a bit unhinged standing there having a good sniff, close to tears.*
>
> *I have been noticing things every day and am really looking forward to the next treatment.*
>
> *Thank you, Dawn*

There is always some reservation after initial success and with Dawn I felt especially apprehensive, but over the next sessions, two to four weeks apart, governed as they were by work commitments and holidays, there was always news of improvement after every visit. Dawn told me she could smell chocolate again! And taste raspberry coulis! Just like the good old days! After her third treatment, she said she felt there was some 'fine-tuning' going on as her list of smells kept growing – apple shampoo, fairy liquid and the contents of the rubbish bag were added!

The biggest change in her was when she could taste her food again, notably her Christmas dinner, unlike the previous year. She had also been dreading going on holiday and not being able to enjoy tasting meals with Jarlath, but she went on holiday after only two sessions and enjoyed every meal. Jarlath told me what a difference it made to him too. Dawn was happier in herself, and when Jarlath cooked their dinners he found it pleasurable again, rather than the chore it had been when Dawn hadn't enjoyed eating. There were downsides for Dawn, though, the biggest of which was being able to smell the wounds of patients again at the GP practice where she worked!

We talked about her concerns that these benefits would regress and her hyposmia would return, but they didn't. What acupuncture probably did for her was rewire the communication between the sensory smell cells in her nose and brain, by stimulating the nerves connecting them. Because smell and taste are inextricably linked it is understandable that acupuncture can help with both. Dawn should be fine now, unless the same situation arises again – a combination of a viral infection and stress to trigger a loss.

Dawn kept on experiencing new smells after each of her four treatments over a two-month period, but none were as dramatic as the changes after her very first session. In fact, there were no more changes after her fifth and sixth treatments so that's when we stopped. Dawn was delighted at that point to have – as she put it – ninety-five per cent of her smelling ability back. This has lasted ever since, despite an upper-respiratory viral infection.

Dawn was my first hyposmia subject, and her case makes me wonder just how many people are out there with little or no sense of smell (or taste) and how they might benefit from acupuncture. Perhaps people with PVOD, without other concurrent diseases like diabetes, Alzheimer's or Parkinson's that can all contribute to a loss of smell, would be best helped by acupuncture. This needs to be investigated further.

I had just received more positive feedback from Dawn in an email when Larissa arrived for acupuncture for her back problems. I had treated her dog Sam over a long time, and Larissa had been coming for her own treatment ever since. I excitedly told her about the initial success with Dawn – anonymously of course, to respect patient confidentiality. Despite many in-depth conversations with Larissa over the years, from suggesting the topic for her degree dissertation on animal diseases caused by Schmallenberg virus, to the state of the planet and her aches and pains, she had never mentioned her decade-long loss of smell. Or if she had, I had forgotten because neither of us had known that acupuncture could help. She was very willing to try it out, but the one treatment had no effect and so I encouraged her to go for medical investigation first.

Then there was Betty who, at 84 years of age, came to me with a poor sense of taste and smell that had persisted for at least six years. She was delighted by the improvement during five acupuncture treatments, although her response was not as spectacular as Dawn's. Unfortunately, after having a fall she was unable to continue treatment.

— 16 —
Stem cells, opiates and acupuncture

The next two cases, one animal and one human, are linked because both had back pain and problems with medication and both came to acupuncture via the veterinary practice. There are always new developments in veterinary and human medicine and there are often parallels between them. You only need to watch the *Supervet* in action on TV to see what complex surgical procedures are available now for our pets and why pet insurance is so important if you want to be able to afford them. But at the time of writing, dogs are ahead of humans in one therapeutic area and that is in the field of stem cell therapy.

At the St Clair practice, orthopaedic vet Ian was innovative in advancing techniques for repairing cruciate ligaments. The latest technique he made available was stem cell therapy for dogs who have painful arthritic joints. Apparently this therapy is in the pipeline for humans in the future, but the animals have beaten us to it. Saying that, for certain conditions it is still classed as experimental.

Stem cell therapy involves harvesting cells under general anaesthesia from a fatty area of the animal's body, such as the shoulder, and the sample is sent to a lab for processing. The stem cells are extracted and concentrated and then injected back into the animal's joint, along with platelet-rich plasma, or PRP. The PRP is prepared at the same time by centrifuging the blood to spin out the platelet cells until they are in a concentrated form. This is analogous to gardening, whereby the stem cells are 'seeds' that are planted in a joint, and the PRP is the 'fertiliser'; together they stimulate repair of the damaged tissue. Here is the story of one particular dog who has benefited from this modern cutting-edge procedure – as well as the ancient therapy of acupuncture which is at least two thousand years old!

Petra the Border Collie—stiffness and stem cells

Petra's first visit to her local vet's practice was at eight weeks of age, for an out-of-hours consultation. She had breathing difficulties that were linked to kennel cough (a viral and bacterial respiratory infection) so, luckily, a course of antibiotic treatment plus a few weeks' rest led to a full recovery. She went back with lameness and stiffness when she was only ten months old. X-rays were taken of her hips and hip dysplasia was ruled out. Like all Border Collies, she was full of beans, which probably meant she would always be prone to overdoing things.

At seven years old, Petra often had stiff hind limbs, but it would ease off with rest and with the anti-inflammatory medication, meloxicam. However, when she was nine, she was out on a walk and suddenly pulled up lame. She could hardly touch the toes of her right back leg on the ground. This prompted a full x-ray examination of her spine, hips and knees. Cruciate ligament rupture seemed the likely culprit because of a forward movement when her knee was manipulated. It was likely she would need surgery to repair it. However, she also had abnormalities of both her kneecaps, which allowed more movement than is normal. The actual problem was a sprained and thickened right Achilles tendon (like ours, this is above the back of the ankle (tarsus) – the equivalent of a dog's hock joint; see Fig. 3). Unfortunately spondylosis was also spotted on the x-rays, affecting several vertebrae from T12 to L7 (see page 60), which was probably the cause of her back pain and stiffness. The abnormal movement of the knees was considered to be due to altered gait because she had to compensate for her back pain. Petra didn't need an operation after all. It was back to conservative treatment – more rest and the addition of gabapentin to keep her comfortable along with her meloxicam.

Petra first underwent the newly offered option of stem cell therapy when an episode of left-hind lameness was linked to inflammation and pain in the tendon below her left kneecap – patellar tendinitis. Her vet Ian subsequently pin-pointed a source of pain at the lumbosacral joint, and she had a second round of stem cell treatment delivered by epidural injection, into her spine. Petra improved on both occasions after a period of rest and medication, but a few months after the second treatment she became very sore again. She had been for a quick paddle and swim in the pond at a local park and the following morning she didn't want to stand up. During that day she sat down to eat and was clearly stiffer after just a little bit of walking. Her owners booked an emergency appointment, where a pain-killing injection was given, then she visited Ian again. When he palpated her back, the area of pain in her spine seemed to have expanded, despite the fact that she was on pain medication and a joint supplement. Ian added tramadol, an opiate, on to her prescription in case it would be needed. Nothing more could be done for her surgically and as she was on the full range of pain-relief medicines, Ian referred her to me for acupuncture. Petra's owner Ellen subsequently commented:

"One of the difficulties through all of this was that at the time, when her pain was the worst, the extra medication needed to manage it partially sedated her, as well as easing her pain, something which neither she nor we were comfortable with. It's also worth noting that Petra lives in a house that has three floors, and level access to the garden is only available from the basement. We had been very grateful for the excellent care that she'd received up to this point, but I must admit the thought of giving her more treatment in the form of acupuncture troubled me. Petra had been through a lot already, and we questioned whether it was right to put her through more – and to be honest we were all a bit weary. Petra seemed to be in pain all the time and, much as she loved walks, they were not comfortable for her. There was also a sense of waiting for something else to go wrong. Because we had run out of options we took Ian's advice to try acupuncture."

I had treated Cello, a Golden Retriever, who responded well to acupuncture. But his owner wanted to do her utmost to give him the best quality of life in the future because he was only three years old. He went off for stem cell therapy and did so well that he didn't need to come back for acupuncture. Both of his elbows had been enlarged – hugely – due to an inherited degenerative joint condition. This is a condition for which stem cell therapy works best, when specific joints are pinpointed as the problem – like Cello's elbows. It is not a cure-all if the animal has multiple joints affected by arthritis or, like Petra, if spondylosis had extended along the spine.

I saw in her notes that Petra had sometimes been so wriggly that the vet needed a nurse to help out during routine examinations, and administering her kennel-cough vaccine was quite a pantomime (it goes up the nose, so it's not surprising many dogs object!). Naturally I wondered how she would react to acupuncture. I didn't need to worry as it turns out; right from the start Petra was totally at home and loved the attention.

The aim of using acupuncture with Petra was to supplement the medication she was already on and see if it would help control her pain better and aid her mobility, especially of her left hind leg. I questioned Ellen at Petra's assessment session. She told me that Petra tired easily when out walking and objected to her back being handled or brushed. Petra yawned and stretched more, which she thought were signs of discomfort. While these aren't common signs of pain, they were something out of the ordinary. This is why owners' observations are so helpful, and they have helped me keep an open mind about what 'normal' is.

Petra settled on the clinic table and while she reacted to almost every needle placed along either side of her spine with a mild muscle twitch, she was quite happy. At the next session, Ellen reported that Petra had been sleepy afterwards. She felt there had been a huge improvement overall – Petra became livelier and happier and was rarely yawning or stretching. She was still a bit stiff in the evenings, but far better again by the next morning. Ellen told me that Petra didn't mind being brushed again – a sure sign that her back wasn't so sore! As before, Petra was happy on the table, so I treated additional points which responded with more twitches as she lay down on her tummy, perfectly relaxed. These were good signs.

Before the third session, Petra had jumped up onto the bed twice, which she hadn't done for ages, and was digging more in the garden. Even so, Ellen thought that she hadn't had such a good week overall. She suggested that Petra had over-exercised, so was becoming stiffer at night, and she was back to yawning and stretching more. Petra was more fidgety during the third treatment, so Ellen and I decided that a week of rest would be helpful. By her fourth visit, she had improved again and she was more relaxed during the acupuncture. We increased the interval to a month as originally planned.

One month later, Ellen described Petra as being more resilient and managing short walks well. Brushing was no problem whatsoever. Another month on and, at her sixth acupuncture treatment, Petra was full of beans again, hardly yawning or stretching, as happy as ever to come in for her treatment and be lifted up onto the table. I was really impressed that Ellen didn't think of Petra as a patient anymore – it was a lovely thought and indicated progress indeed! Ellen summarised our journey with Petra in an email.

From the first acupuncture treatment the improvement in Petra's con-dition was very obvious. The constant yawning and stretching that had become the norm when Petra was in pain almost disappeared and she

> *was clearly more energised and livelier. Over time I stopped worrying that her pain was unmanageable and actually enjoyed taking her for walks again, albeit much shorter ones than previously.*
>
> *That's not to say there haven't been episodes of increased stiffness and pain – Jane has been very honest that we are 'fighting the ageing process'. But we have had long periods of consistency and Petra has been on the same dose of medication (with occasional increases and extra rest) for some time at a level that does not sedate her.*
>
> *The acupuncture also appears to have achieved a level of resilience in Petra's condition that has surprised me. There have been episodes where I have been concerned that a worsening of her condition was permanent, only to have her improve again over time.*
>
> *And finally, sometimes it feels as though the benefits of Petra's acupuncture treatment extend a bit beyond the dog herself. With Petra on a table, on a level with us all, and with such a tactile treatment involving us all being hands-on, there is definitely the sense of a communal experience.*

Petra's acupuncture continues every six weeks. Sometimes she can lay her head on Ellen's shoulder and is very chilled throughout her treatment; now and again she is fidgety. Occasionally, after having a 'bigger' day out, Ellen gives Petra one tramadol, but overall her *joie de vivre* is back. Recently Ellen watched helplessly from a distance as Petra climbed a grassy bank and rolled about the body of a dead rat! While she is keener to go on walks, she can tire easily at times and her left hind leg sometimes stiffens up. This is most likely due to developing osteoarthritis in her slightly enlarged knee. When she is taken on longer trips to the beach, it can take a couple of days for the stiffness to go, but Ellen thinks that's a fair trade-off for Petra enjoying a dog's life. She continues to jump on and off the bed, and is happy being brushed. Petra is calmer with other dogs around, too, and Ellen is less worried about how Petra will react to them.

"Life changing," Ellen said, putting into simple words how she describes the effect of acupuncture.

Meanwhile, vet Ian is convinced that without acupuncture Petra would be on a high dose of painkillers for back pain and the side effects would adversely affect her quality of life. He also says that in the future, when treating an older dog, he will consider trying acupuncture before using stem cell therapy – but we both agree that Petra has had the best of both worlds.

Craig's back pain—electro-acupuncture

As Ellen doesn't drive, her neighbour Craig had brought her and Petra to the practice and accompanied them during treatments. After a few discussions of Petra's progress, as well as acupuncture in general, for both animals and people, Craig started to talk about his back. As one of Petra's dog walkers, he was mightily impressed by her response and asked me about acupuncture for himself.

He had a complicated history. Chronic spinal-nerve pain had forced him to stop working four years earlier and some years before that, when he was just in his mid-thirties, he had multiple episodes of deep vein thrombosis (DVT) in his leg. This is where blood clots form that block some blood vessels, an excruciatingly painful condition which can be life-threatening if the clots travel to the lungs or the brain. Craig was on a life-long prescription for warfarin to keep his blood thin and prevent further clots developing. At one time the warfarin had been stopped but he had suffered a second DVT six months later.

At the time, Craig was undergoing a course of acupuncture at the hospital pain clinic to help with his inoperable spinal condition. He had two out of three planned sessions and found it to be relaxing, and enjoyed the great night's sleep that followed. While he was lying down for his third session, however, the specialist acupuncture nurse spotted and correctly diagnosed the second DVT in his leg, and thereafter acupuncture was ruled out – at that time there were concerns that it may have caused bleeding and clots to form, given that he had not been on warfarin. Thus began his life of daily warfarin and continued pain medication and wearing compression stockings. He had benefited from attending an NHS Pain Clinic with its multidisciplinary approach including self-help techniques, but felt he had plateaued. He was stuck, so was now wondering about acupuncture again.

I had suggested to him that he should speak to his GP about the possibility of getting acupuncture treatment for back pain through the NHS, but the next time he came in with Petra he looked crestfallen. His GP had completely denigrated acupuncture although he was quite happy to give repeat prescriptions of the pain medications gabapentin, tramadol and amitriptyline, along with paracetamol. Tramadol is an opiate and Craig wanted to avoid it. He'd been hooked on it before, taking increasing doses until they had a major impact on his daily life, affecting his thought processes without alleviating his pain.

While his doctor said he wouldn't refer him for acupuncture he didn't say there were any reasons why he shouldn't have it, healthwise. However he assumed that, because needles were involved, it could be ruled out because Craig was taking warfarin. When the phlebotomist took Craig's next blood sample to measure his warfarin level, she assured him there was no reason for him not to have acupuncture. He had been on warfarin for ten years since his DVT and his clotting factors were stable (the unit for measuring blood-clotting ability is the INR, meaning International Normalized Ratio). It wasn't safe for Craig to take certain anti-inflammatories like aspirin and ibuprofen for his pain because they would react with the warfarin, but according to the BMAS guidelines it was safe for him to try acupuncture. Carefully placed small-gauge needles should do no harm.

In January 2019, Craig duly came for his first treatment at the medical surgery where I saw my human patients. He shared more details of his history. After hospital investigations, multiple bulging discs in his lower lumbar region had been diagnosed as the cause of his severe spinal pain. There had been no sign of degeneration or trauma and there was no surgical option, the discs had simply dried out and were pressing on the nerves that exited nearby.

He told me he was coping with sciatica in his left leg, where pain travels down the length of the sciatic nerve. Five years before that, he had had a very painful 'frozen' shoulder. Craig knew all about pain and the impact it had had on his life – he'd been forced to give up his accountancy work four years earlier because of it. As he desperately wanted to avoid the side effects of medication as much as possible, he was often left struggling with the pain. He was trying to manage on paracetamol alone, taking up to the maximum dose of eight a day, and only taking the stronger painkillers when absolutely necessary. He wanted to be able to support his wife and four teenage children in their daily lives as best he could. As a former cyclist he still tried to go to the gym regularly but had to be careful because of the changes in his spine. He could easily get cramp-like feelings in his leg because the blood supply was reduced, as his consultant explained, due to the veins in his leg failing to reopen fully following the DVTs.

For Craig's first treatment I planned a minimal approach using acupuncture without massage, and starting with pain and back points, because I had no idea how sensitive he would be. I included points on the whole of his back, not just the base where he felt pain, and I found the muscles were so solid that his back was like a wooden board! The feedback Craig gave during that first session was a good indication that he was sensitive to acupuncture. He was aware of a feeling of 'muscle tremor' with some needles, especially around his shoulder.

"It was like a weight lifted off my shoulders that I hadn't realised was there," he was pleased to report. This was followed shortly after by an intense sensation of relaxation. "A bit like a Ready-Brek glow!' he said. He had a deep feeling of calmness and a very deep sleep that night.

At the second session, two weeks later, I started with massage, which Craig found very relaxing. This time, however, he didn't get the 'Ready-Brek glow'. Instead he felt worn out and didn't do much for the rest of the day, and went to bed early. He did sleep well, though, and the following day he went to his exercise class. "It felt much easier, as if my joints had been greased and cycling felt effortless," he reported.

Because Craig had such a chronic condition and had coped well with treatment so far, at his third visit, one month later, I introduced electro-acupuncture for a stronger effect and because of its known usefulness for treating chronic pain. He found the sensation caused by the pulsing current through the needles somewhat strange but reported that two hours later, back at home, he felt profoundly relaxed and calm both physically and mentally – a state that he had previously only experienced with a full-blown mix of medication with gabapentin, amitriptyline and tramadol. The effect lasted most of the day and he was very tired, although, as he explained, he had the beginnings of a cold. He slept well again and the relaxant effect easily lasted for forty-eight hours. Unfortunately, his cold worsened and five days later he had to visit another GP who prescribed antibiotics. Craig mentioned the acupuncture to this second doctor and was again met with dismissal. The doctor said he could try it if he wanted, but it would probably do no good, and he expected it should be excluded anyway because of his ongoing warfarin treatment.

Another month later, Craig was keen to continue, despite finding the electro-acupuncture to be a bit uncomfortable at his last visit. This time he said it wasn't as uncomfortable – 'just a little irritating'. "I was aware of a faint buzzing/drilling-type sensation," he later told me, "but it was much less intrusive and I was less aware once all the needles were in place with the currents going at the same time seeming to cancel each other out". Immediately after that session, he felt very tired and chilled out, describing it as 'a lowered state of awareness'. He had kept the window of the car down while driving home, explaining "As if relaxed but exhausted after some kind of endurance exercise."

The tiredness lasted for a few days but he slept better and longer throughout the nights with uninterrupted spells of sleep of up to seven hours. The tiredness was even worse one Saturday night when he stayed up late. "I felt massively fatigued for forty-eight hours after, but then I was surprised to feel more switched on and more able to exercise with good effort at the gym!"

The following month, at the fifth session of electro-acupuncture followed by massage, Craig reported that he didn't feel as tired straight after, just more relaxed and chilled. He slept very soundly again, and had much deeper sleeps for up to seven hours at a time for four nights after the treatment. He reported back, "I'm consistently now experiencing a powerful relaxant effect similar to opiate or nerve-pain suppressant drugs previously prescribed."

At the sixth session, the same treatment was given. Craig coped with a stronger electric current that stimulated twitches in his left shoulder muscles. "By seven o'clock that night," he said, "I felt a lightness across my shoulders and freer movement in my arms – like adding oil to a taut chain. When walking, around nine pm, my shoulders felt almost weightless – as if a weight had been pressing on them before and just been removed. This overall feeling also translated generally to reduced stress and a calm, relaxed disposition. I went cycling for the first time in a while. I slept longer and better post-acupuncture, including a full seven hours straight on the night of the treatment. Markedly, I noticed my shoulders were easier and less tense at the gym after acupuncture." Craig's benefits from combined acupuncture and massage were:

- He consistently experienced a powerful relaxant effect similar to when he took the opiate and nerve-pain suppressant before, and is coping well on three to four paracetamol a day. If he has a flare-up, usually for some lifestyle reason, he takes more, perhaps six or seven a day. He has never felt the need for stronger medication since beginning the treatment.

- Overall, his movements feel easier and his mobility has increased.

- Before he was waking up every two to three hours, but now he usually sleeps for five or six hours, sometimes seven, and when he was on holiday he was amazed to wake up after ten hours.

- There was a positive effect on his general health and well-being, and he is riding his bike again after a gap of eighteen months.

Craig still comes for his monthly appointments and Petra is having six-weekly sessions. Both are doing well.

A little update about Petra

In October 2019, when she was twelve and a half, Petra had her right eye removed. She had glaucoma, where the eye enlarges due to fluid building up, causing high pressure inside the eye that can be painful. Conservative treatment helped to control it for a while, but it only delayed the inevitable. It was a tough time for Ellen and the family when the decision to operate had to be made, but Petra totally surprised them. After a few days wearing a buster collar to stop her rubbing the wound, normality resumed. Petra can see well with just her left eye and the right eye space is surrounded by black fur – you can barely notice the difference.

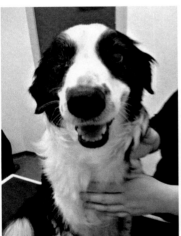 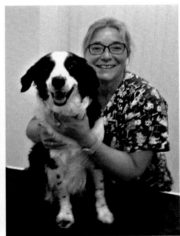

Petra is happy, despite losing her right eye; enjoying a cuddle with me (right).

Analgesics and acupuncture

I have been lucky so far. Personally, I have had no need for strong painkillers so I have no experience of their effects, but I am reminded of the effect on a client's wife. Bill, a retired policeman, always had some interesting stories to tell while we treated his dog Cass. He became very animated, telling me of one day in the previous week when his wife had become unwell after having driven from Fife to her workplace in Edinburgh. She was unable to drive home so Bill had collected her. Her GP visited as soon as she got home because she was feeling so strange. On close questioning he ascertained that Ann had in fact taken Cass's tramadol tablet by mistake – she stored her own and Cass's tablets in the same drawer. Her GP was less than impressed but I breathed a sigh of relief on behalf of the practice that it was not a veterinary mistake; all of Cass's medications were clearly labelled with her name and address, the drug's name and the dosage.

It seems a mystery that some people can still have such closed minds to acupuncture when it may be, for some, an alternative to strong medication that can affect mental capacity and wreak havoc on their lives. It is well-known that the UK is one of many societies that have a huge problem with analgesic dependency for many people living with chronic pain. Craig alerted me to information he gleaned at the regular self-help pain-management group he attends: that Fife is the NHS region in Scotland with the highest use of prescription painkillers.

At that time, in May 2019, I asked my GP friend Liz about it.

"We are doing our very best in a difficult situation," she sighed. "With the lack of resources there is little alternative at present in our area – it's a twenty-six-week wait for physiotherapy and a twelve-month wait for a pain clinic appointment".

This situation is certainly not conducive to lessening the dependency on pain medication. When the subject of pain management came up at an acupuncture meeting not long after Liz's comment, an NHS nurse said that in 2018 funding had been withdrawn for her acupuncture clinic. She deals with patients who are in chronic pain who have been through the range of investigations and treatments offered by the NHS and have ended up on increasing levels of opiates. While the regulations permitted only six sessions per patient before discharge (and some ideally needed continuous treatment), the acupuncture allowed many of them to reduce their drug use and improve their quality of life; but it was no longer available to them. She was hoping to work privately to provide what she sees as an invaluable service, but it may still be unavailable for those who cannot afford to pay – and she hopes the NHS regulations will change again in the future to make acupuncture an option for her pain patients.

The question is, just how many 'Craigs' are out there suffering from unmanageable chronic pain – who would benefit from acupuncture?

— 17 —

Tales of the unexpected (including the case of the twitching buttocks)

At the heart of science is an essential balance between two seemingly contra-dictory attitudes – an openness to new ideas, no matter how bizarre or coun-terintuitive they may be – and the most ruthless sceptical scrutiny of all ideas, old and new. This is how deep truths are winnowed from deep nonsense.

Carl Sagan *(American astrophysicist)*

As I tried to draw this book to a conclusion in May 2019, which marked my twenty years practising acupuncture, new interesting cases kept coming up that I felt I just couldn't leave out. In his book, *A Life in Questions*, Jeremy Paxman says:

> *The real reason people write is that they feel they must, it is not to make a living ... On days when it goes well it is like surfing, on bad days it is like trying to swim in treacle.*

I can identify with this. I find I can 'surf' best from memory, but when my memories are not too accurate – when the treacle appears – then I rely on my clinical histories. In this Chapter I indulged in a bit of 'surfing' through my more recent interactions with people and experiences, so it contains quite a mixed bag of events and cases.

October 2018—vet reunion in Glasgow

Thirty-five years after qualifying from vet school, my ex-university friends and I met up. We mingled around the tables in a function room of the Grosvenor Hotel in the West End of Glasgow as the decibels of our voices increased during the evening, until we could hardly hear the background music. It was a wonderful atmosphere. What a mixed bag we were! Some of our number had already retired from practice, many of whom had sold their business to large corporate organisations when the profession had begun to change; so very different from the days of James Herriot. Alf Wight – the real James Herriot – was also a Glasgow graduate and I went through my teens reading his books, but experiencing mixed practice in Fife had dispelled many illusions

I once had about what life as a vet would be like. The reality involved long hours, tough decisions and mountains of responsibility.

We recalled, at that reunion, how 1978 had been the second year in which the number of female students had equalled the number of males. Historically, there was a better chance of getting on to the course if you played rugby and were the son of a farmer or a vet. Nowadays, seventy to eighty per cent of the students are female. The number of Scottish students is much lower nowadays, as other nationalities arrive from all over the world. And now you have to provide an elaborate CV and a personal statement, on top of having top exam grades, to stand a chance of getting in – my three As and two Bs at Higher level were valued at the time, but would be scoffed at today.

There were only sixty-nine of us in my year, excluding the single student who left the course after just two days. Another one of us transferred to medicine after two years, and one didn't qualify at the end of the five years. Around six of us went off to the Antipodes – never to return to work in the UK. A few left the profession quite early. Teresa, for instance, went on to have a long career working in all aspects of food safety with a local council, where her training in veterinary microbiology came in very handy. Eleanor spent a career in vet practice, and – five children later – retrained as a music teacher. Several others once owned, and still own, very successful small-animal practices.

Some of my classmates had become the owners of equine, bovine and mixed practices. One became Dean of Liverpool vet school, another a senior Home Office Inspector, and Mark Johnston became the most successful racehorse trainer in British racing history (in August 2018), while keeping his veterinary surgeon registration. He says his veterinary background gave him a very different perspective on caring for and training racehorses.

Two of my fellow students specialised in alternative therapies, training in homeopathy and acupuncture, and another couple of them used acupuncture in their practices (although there may have been more). Carol was one such vet, and told me how super-pulsed laser therapy largely superseded her use of acupuncture.

When I was newly qualified, I had thought I would join a mixed practice, for both farm and small animals, but I had to re-sit one of my exams which delayed my entry into the veterinary world. There were fewer jobs around then and so – being female – it was small-animal practice for me. At that point I had no idea how varied my career would be, or that I would work Down Under, or that I would spend at least twenty years practising acupuncture.

November 2018—vet acupuncture clinic in Glenrothes

One morning, Kevin, my first veterinary client of the day, asked me, "So what are you up to?".

He was a regular sponsor of my charity sporting activities and was expecting some kind of sporty news, but as things had quietened down for the winter I told him there wasn't much to report, just a 10K run the following month that I wasn't training enough for. However, there was another thing I was feeling very unsure about, and my guilty secret slipped out, hesitantly. "Well" I told him, "I'm planning to write a book, about acupuncture – and I'm thinking of putting you in it!"

He said as long I portrayed him as a George Clooney-esque figure, he didn't mind me writing about his dog, Flora; not that he was expecting her to be in the book – but of course she is, and he is (although I didn't dwell on the George Clooney aspect!).

That day is vividly etched in my memory because of the combination of events that unfolded, which demonstrate why practising as both a vet and acupuncturist is so meaningful to me. A boxed gift and a card had been handed in by Wilma, a retired minister, who had so often brought her dog Gabby to see me. Cheryl and I had the reception area to ourselves briefly. She cried as she read out Wilma's words on the card, words that thanked me for the gift of acupuncture and what it had done for Gabby, until she was put to sleep. I held myself together until I saw that the box contained a Willowtree figurine called the 'angel of healing'. I can't tell you how touched I was. It is very humbling when you feel the depth of someone's emotion for their animal friend, and the yawning gap they leave behind. We had often talked about how Gabby just kept going, despite her bandy legs, and how she loved coming to me for acupuncture. I felt sad, but then I braced myself for the day that lay ahead.

Border Collie Petra (who you met in Chapter 16) was my next patient, pulling hard on her lead as ever, desperate to come into the consulting room. She had completed her initial course of four acupuncture sessions, and her owner Ellen told me that Petra was doing really well. That was rewarding. Craig (also from Chapter 16), who had driven them to the practice that day, agreed with her, but went on to tell me that his GP had pooh-poohed his request for acupuncture for his back pain, and had instead given him another prescription, for four different drugs. As you can imagine, I was dismayed to hear this. Then, later that day, I met up with my GP friend, Liz. She told me about some alarming new evidence that had been published in the press that morning, about a link between certain painkillers and sudden death. We discussed how current treatment protocols can limit the choices of people who are really suffering. In her opinion – and, of course, in mine too – acupuncture should be considered more for the management of pain. It is *always* worth trying – and what an outcome it is when someone can reduce their medications, or come off tablets altogether, and avoid all their inherent side effects.

In between my other appointments, Susan – the owner of Labrador Skye – called me. She sounded upset and my first thoughts were about her dog, that something had happened to her. But Susan assured me that Skye was fine. She was actually looking for an appointment for herself, to help with her sore back. She laughed out loud when I said, "Oh, that's alright then!". I was referring to the fact that it was her who had the problem, not Skye, but my words didn't come out the way I wanted them to. She knew I wasn't implying that she was less important than her pet!

Later on, I clipped Dachshund Otto's nails. His owner couldn't bear to look. Otto was a bit of a wriggler and she found the procedure more worrying than the acupuncture he'd just had for his back. How very differently we view interventions!

It was a thought-provoking day, and by the end of it I realised how deeply satisfying it was to work with acupuncture; how right and enjoyable it was to be able to treat both pets and their owners. So often they had the same needs, yet so many people have never heard what acupuncture can do for them, let alone the possibility of treating their pets, who might even like it! I thought seriously that day about recording some of my experiences, and that is how this book came about.

December 2018—10K run in Tillicoultry

The sun was shining and it was ten degrees Celsius outside – positively balmy for the end of December in Scotland. I had only signed up for the run because my nieces were doing it too, and because two months earlier I suspected I would need motivation to keep training. They had done their best with me, but I had let things slip and hardly ran at all in preparation for the race. And I'd put on weight. The Half Ironman I had done the previous August felt like a very long time ago.

Nieces Karyn and Diane were also feeling under-prepared (if not as much as their aunty), and I was swept along by their enthusiasm to get running. The fact I had arrived at the start-line *at all* was some achievement! They were forfeiting their usual Saturday morning park run in Dunfermline to take part in this event, the Tillicoultry 10K. What a setting it was! The clear blue sky outlined the nearby Ochil Hills, which rose from road level to over two thousand feet. We would be running along the foothills by the cycle-way, and it was going to be dry but windy.

There was little time to hang around. The instructions were given then we were off, along with another three hundred or so runners. A constant stream of them passed me by and I knew I'd be very near the end. My plan was to jog halfway, then do a joggy-walk back from the turn-around point and so get to the finish in one piece. So I plodded on. Just keep going, I thought. I checked my watch after eighteen minutes as the lead runner came towards me at an amazing speed – already on his return trip. I found out later he had run in the Commonwealth Games! Don't let it bother you, I told myself. One step at a time …

The occasional person still overtook me and I knew I must be near to last. I was aware of a beeping sound behind me, which got fainter then louder again. I assumed it was another runner's electronic pacer, changing in loudness as the distance between us varied. Arriving at the halfway drinking station, I found the 'beeper' beside me. We struck up a conversation and she introduced herself as Jill. I had decided to take a breather, but perhaps, when I got going again, I could try to match her routine and keep going alongside her, with the beeping leading the way. Jill explained that it timed her so that she ran for forty seconds then walked for twenty. I mentioned my idea and she was delighted to have the company because she had been struggling too. So we set off together.

I had no idea how fortuitous this meeting would turn out to be. Jill intrigued me from the start, not just because I noticed she was wearing earrings made by my favourite designer, Sheila Fleet. We chatted all the way to the finish line. As Jill's story about herself unfolded, she made a deep impression on me. She had been on crutches for three years after an accident in which a car had collided with hers. Two knee operations later, her surgeons told her that they doubted she would ever walk again. But before the accident Jill had been a Scottish International rugby player – and a firefighter. She was made of tough stuff.

She sounded like an expert in rehab with all she'd been through, but there was more that afflicted her. She had been hospitalised on more than one occasion with allergic reactions to the drugs that were prescribed for her. It was then discovered that she had Stevens–Johnson syndrome, which I had never heard of before. It's a rare disease that becomes a medical emergency when the body's reaction to medication or an infection causes serious damage to the skin and mucous linings.

Yet, despite all these setbacks, she had still managed to run three marathons! It was jaw-dropping stuff. Then she told me she had tried acupuncture and it had transformed her life. She had started it with a traditionally trained acupuncturist earlier that year and was going for treatment every two or three weeks. The constant pain she had experienced in her knee for fifteen years disappeared. The debility she experienced because of her knee, and the days off work she had taken as a result of her endometriosis, had reduced to a manageable level. She told me she wished she had known about acupuncture years ago.

It goes without saying that Jill inspired me enormously, and she sealed my commitment to writing up these tales about the role of acupuncture in both human and veterinary medicine. We share the hope that this book spreads the word about acupuncture far and wide.

January 2019—Edinburgh Zoo

My husband Kenneth and I took a trip to the zoo one day, because we had never seen the pandas. I didn't understand why the pandas were brought to Scotland in the first place, so distant from their natural environment, with their specific nutritional and habitat requirements, and as for the cost … But I have to admit it was amazing to see them close up. On a plaque outside their enclosure was a quotation by Confucius:

Real knowledge is to know the extent of one's ignorance.

These simple words struck a chord with me, especially about how little I still knew about acupuncture and how it actually works. There is a point near the wrist called PC6, which stops nausea and sickness by some debated mechanism. I still wonder whether acupuncture would have prevented Nicola's fate, who I was to hear about in the Spring of 2019. You will read about her a little later in this chapter.

February 2019—Dawn's consultant

Dawn (who I talked about in Chapter15) was so delighted to have her sense of smell and taste back that she wrote to her ENT hospital consultant about it. Her story piqued his interest so much that he wanted to meet up with GP Liz and I to find out more. He dropped into Millhill Surgery, where we were both working as he was passing between hospitals. Liz had been happy to be treated with the same points I used on Dawn – they had helped her hay fever! The three of us discussed the possibility that acupuncture needles had stimulated Dawn's olfactory nerve and its connections, allowing them to function again. The ENT consultant wanted to carry out a clinical trial to see whether some of his NHS patients, who had no apparent cause for their anosmia and hyposmia, despite exhaustive tests, would benefit from acupuncture. The problem was, the best test kits for assessing a person's ability to smell before and after treatment were expensive, and there was no funding available. Without obtaining robust knowledge, the results wouldn't stand up as 'evidence' that would be taken seriously. So yet another wonderful opportunity was going by the wayside.

March 2019—-the Association of British Veterinary Acupuncturists Conference, Birmingham

I sat through a full morning of lectures given by a doctor called Dan Keown. He is a British-trained medical doctor who also has a degree in Chinese acupuncture and has visited experts in China to learn more. He has written two books on the subject, namely *The Spark in the Machine* (2013) and *The Uncharted Body* (2018). His aim is to bridge the gap between Chinese acupuncture and Western medical acupuncture, convinced as he is that both systems complement each other. His talks were fascinating and included descriptions on the relation between the Chinese channels and anatomical development of the embryo. There was a lot to take on board and I thought of acupuncture vet, Ann, who always said that studying both branches of acupuncture had led her to seeing health and disease in a different, more enlightened way.

Afterwards, I asked Dan for some advice. I told him I was trying to write a book about treating animals and people with acupuncture, but that I wasn't going to include references to the medical literature – something that might be frowned upon. He simply said:

"Just write! Just do it!"

April 2019—Nicola's tardive dyskinesia

I had never heard of tardive dyskinesia until I met Nicola, who I mentioned earlier. She was a GP and had been diagnosed with the condition by a neurologist. It wasn't good news. According to the *Oxford Concise Medical Dictionary*, the condition is:

> *... characterized by involuntary repetitive movements of the facial muscles and the tongue, usually resembling continued chewing motions, and the muscles of the limbs. It is associated with long-term medication with certain anti-psychotic drugs, especially the phenothiazines, and occurs predominantly in older patients, particularly women.*

Phenothiazines are a group of chemically related compounds that have various pharmacological actions – they are used as anti-psychotics as well as worming and anti-sickness medications. Because this type of drug affects different systems in the body, they have many possible side effects.

I had first met Nicola at the end of 2018, when she came to me for acupuncture. She thought several of her symptoms – the teeth clenching, the choking sensation, the pressure at the front of her neck, and her neck pain – might be related to the extensive dental work she'd had done previously. Her symptoms were confusing, and after three sessions of acupuncture with me, they showed no improvement. She had already seen a gastroenterologist who'd carried out an endoscopy, where a tube with a camera is passed via the oesophagus into the stomach to look for something wrong. Her results had been normal. Then she saw a neurologist, and that is when she texted me in January, to tell me she'd been diagnosed with tardive dyskinesia.

So three months after her diagnosis, I bumped into her in the changing rooms of our local gym. Her condition had worsened. She had been hospitalised again, and signed off work indefinitely. The tardive dyskinesia had been caused by an anti-sickness medication she'd been taking. It contained prochlorperazine, one of the phenothiazines. These tablets can be bought over the counter at any pharmacy, and Nicola wants people to know about this recognised side effect – which is why I am including her experience in this book.

As I said, I hadn't been able to help Nicola with her neurological symptoms, but around a year after meeting her at the gym I received this update:

> *After 10 months' off work I am mostly recovered. I am only occasionally aware of throat and tongue spasms but fortunately no one notices. I stopped taking prochlorperazine 18 months ago. As a GP I am now very much aware of possible significant side-effects of 'simple' non-prescription anti-sickness tablets that are sold by pharmacies in the UK.*

It leaves me wondering whether, if Nicola had tried acupuncture instead of the medication for her nausea problem, this whole scenario could have been avoided.

May 2019—Hugs from Yana again

I had a breakthrough one day, which was accompanied by a big sigh of relief and an even bigger smile from Rita when she visited with her dog, Yana. Yana made a half-hearted attempt to jump up onto her hind legs, and failed, but the second time she managed it. She put her paws on my chest and looked into my face.

"Now I know she's back to normal" Rita said, as I enjoyed my lovely hug with Yana (pictured *overpage*).

Yana was a very special dog – a ten-year-old Golden Retriever who could still manage to stand up on just her two hind legs. Orthopaedic vet Ian's skills had been needed to repair both of her cruciate ligaments, with operations only three months apart.

She had healed well, but had come back for a course of acupuncture after her recovery period, and after Ian had signed her off from any further check-ups. Gabapentin was the drug that suited her best as she recovered, and for the ongoing pain caused by the spondylosis in her spine.

However Rita had felt she was not yet back to her old self. Despite all of Ian's handiwork, she felt something was not quite right. He had laughed when Rita said, "She needs to see Jane."!

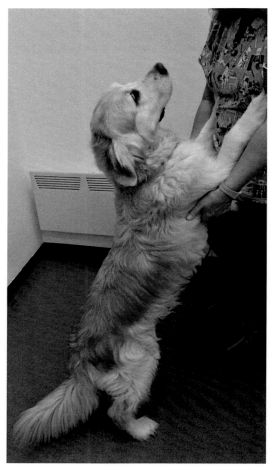

A hug from Yana – able to take her weight on her hind legs once more.

That day, when she came to me with Yana, she knew she had done the right thing. Yana was back to her old self, and that hug she asked for meant a great deal to both of us.

Working with acupuncture for so long has brought families to me for treatment of several of their pets. Rita's family was like Pat and Oscar's (in Chapters 3 and 11 of circling the dragon fame). Rita and I reminisced that day about her three Golden Retrievers that I had treated, and how different they'd all been; one of those three, Star, had received acupuncture from vet John, then me, for a total of ten and a half years. Rita was already familiar with veterinary acupuncture when

I first met her. The St Clair vet, John, had been treating nine-year-old Star for five years, since 2002. Star's history was not straightforward. She had a heart murmur that was detected when she was a pup, but luckily it never caused any problems throughout her life. However, at just over two years of age, she became intolerant to exercise, meaning she was reluctant to run around and struggled to get onto her hind legs after lying down. She was like an old dog. Thorough investigations were carried out at the Dick vet school but they drew a blank, as did subsequent investigations with an orthopaedic veterinary specialist. With nothing to see on her x-rays, the suspected diagnosis was early-stage spondylosis, before bony changes had occurred. The anti-inflammatory drug Metacam™ had helped to some extent, but both John and Rita found that acupuncture helped her even more. Getting into the car and climbing stairs became easier for her, and she also enjoyed and got further benefit from hydrotherapy at a local centre.

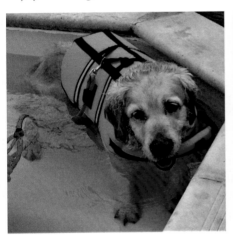 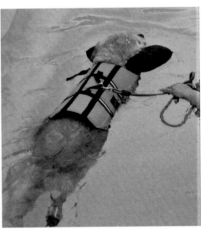

Star in the hydrotherapy pool.

I took over Star's acupuncture treatment when John retired. Acupuncture is not often started in such a young dog, but Star lived a long time, until she was nearly fifteen.

Rita's other dog at that time, Briagha, was different again. She never needed regular acupuncture. As a youngster she suffered acute pain after twisting her back while running on the beach, and simple rest and injection of a painkiller had sorted her out. Briagha was also a show dog, and was entered into the obedience competitions at Crufts.

The event was only two weeks away and Rita didn't want to take any chances, so Briagha paid a visit to John. He treated her back just the once because he hadn't found any signs of pain. She made a full recovery in time to compete.

The next acupuncture request from Rita was unusual. Briagha was not responding as usual to the commands she gave her – could acupuncture help? The answer was, of course, that I had no idea! When Briagha was asked to 'sit' and 'stay', she would paddle with her front legs and sink to the floor – not ideal during an obedience competition. Rita suspected there was some anxiety involved. With nothing to lose I chose acupuncture points to help with relaxation and to relax the muscles around her thoracic spine and shoulders.

Sometime later, Rita reported that Briagha had duly completed four unbroken 'sit and stay' commands over two days of a competition. My naysayer's eyebrows were raised high! Then seven months later Rita made the same request, and the outcome after acupuncture was equally successful. We both remain unsure what happened there, what it was all about, but sometimes there is little point questioning these things if they work!

It was just a natural progression for Yana to come for acupuncture as far as Rita was concerned, especially as it had been such an important part of Star's treatment for that long, long time. At the age of only three, Yana's x-rays revealed spondylosis in her spine so vet Ian recommended acupuncture. It suited Yana down to the ground. Before long, her visits for treatment were a special trip. She was always desperate to come into the consulting room and before I knew it she had her front paws on my chest. After we hug, she lies on the floor (pictured *opposite*), relaxed but keeping watch. If I stop patting her head in between placing a needle, she turns around to nudge me to continue.

July 2019—"Can you treat me?"

"Can the vet that made Bronya better, treat me?" asked the father of Bronya's owner, Sandra. He was eighty-five years old and had a sore neck, but was otherwise fit and still loved swimming. Sandra suspected that the copious lengths of breaststroke – turtle-style – were not helping his neck. I advised he should first have a check-up with his GP and also ask if acupuncture was available to him.

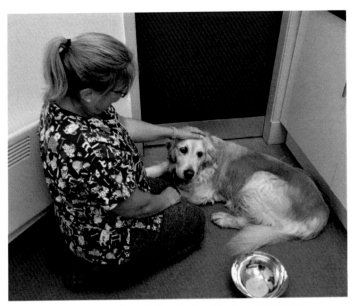

Yana wants to be patted on the head during acupuncture.

Sandra is a veterinary nurse, and has become a great advocate for acupuncture because of the progress she saw in the animals attending the St Clair clinic, including her own Rottweiler, Bronya. Bronya was somewhat unlucky and overall quite a challenging case for the vets who saw her. She was only a year old when she was diagnosed as being 'atopic', that is being super-sensitive to allergy-provoking substances in the environment. This allergic hypersensitivity to many things affected her badly. Her eyes and ears would become irritated, her skin would break out in patches of eczema, and lick granulomas would develop on her paws. Sandra relied on antihistamines and steroids to control the symptoms.

Bronya also often had a seriously upset digestive tract, with vomiting and diarrhoea that made her miserable. Investigations of her blood samples, plus anaesthetics and endoscopies led to a diagnosis of pancreatitis and irritable bowel disease as the cause. Her long-term use of steroids was also damaging her liver. With all this going on, the ageing Bronya grew stiffer and had difficulty walking. Finding an effective medication that would help her without giving her side effects was a problem. Meloxicam caused her to vomit and have diarrhoea, and the opiate tramadol made her even more lethargic and 'not herself'. Acupuncture for her back and hind legs worked a treat. Bronya growled occasionally during her sessions, but this was not related to having a needle placed, and she became very relaxed during the treatments.

Sandra believes that the acupuncture kept Bronya comfortable and was literally a life-saver when there were no pharmaceutical options. On several occasions after treatment, Bronya would stride out along the beach with a plastic bottle in her mouth. That was Sandra's measure of success – when Bronya was feeling her best she would carry that bottle, and with the acupuncture she had gone on carrying her bottle more often than Sandra had anticipated.

August 2019—"Is there nothing else I can do?"

Lesley was a young mum with two young children. She'd had a headache for six painful weeks, and when she had asked her GP "Is there nothing else I can do?', acupuncture was suggested.

What a bad twelve years she'd had! Recurring migraines and headaches at their worst could last for three days. The pain was mostly behind her eyes and she felt sick every half hour or so. Lesley was using four medications in sequence as the severity of the pain progressed – paracetamol, then aspirin, then ibuprofen and then rizatriptan (for acute migraines). She found that if she increased the doses there was less effect, plus the added complication of rebound headaches if she stopped taking the medication. Further investigations and an MRI scan of her brain had all been clear.

Lesley was aware that she often had neck and shoulder pain before a headache struck, and occasionally she felt a lump at the back of her head. She felt better if she stretched her neck out. She worked full-time, sitting at home on her computer for as much as ten hours a day, which all added up to a typical pattern I've seen regularly ever since the days of Bryan and David back in Chapter 5. It didn't help that her computer was on the kitchen table and she sat on an uncomfortable chair, rather than in her office, all because she was keeping company with a new puppy who wanted constant attention!

Before I started any treatment, I was hopeful that I might find some tight muscles – but at the same time I hoped she hadn't been suffering all this time for something as simple as muscle tension. Sure enough, Lesley's cervical and trapezius muscles felt brick-hard, and very tender even with gentle massage. I used a combination of acupuncture points and trigger points. Two weeks after that treatment she told me she'd only had two 'minor' headaches, as she put it, because they didn't stop her activities and medication helped relieve the pain. Her muscles had relaxed considerably.

On my advice, Lesley had been 'air swimming' – standing up and pretending she was swimming, going through the motions of breaststroke, front crawl and backstroke. She found it easier to fit in to her busy lifestyle, and more effective than physiotherapy exercises, as long as she avoided a 'forward head' posture. She had started setting an alarm for regular intervals to get her up out of her seat and away from the computer. I also suggested that she got her pup used to being left alone after his morning walk, settled in his bed, while she worked in her office again. This would prevent him from developing separation anxiety and get Lesley back on her well-designed desk chair!

Lesley asked me whether I saw many cases like hers, and I was sorry to tell her that I did. When I gave her Chapter 5 of this book to read, about headaches, she was amazed at the similarities. She is a textbook case in the acupuncture world – yet not in conventional medicine. She is still having treatment and it continues to make a huge difference to her. Along with changing her routines and exercising, Lesley has been able to increase the intervals between massage and acupuncture treatments. I am sure she is one of countless people who would benefit from massage and acupuncture.

September 2019—Park run

Lewis was easy to spot from a distance. He is always so much taller than the runners around him. He gave me one of his warm hello's and told me how much he enjoyed reviewing my chapter on circling the dragons. Then he bombarded me with questions. I couldn't answer them all. At that time, he was due to enter his final year of veterinary medicine at the Dick vet school – he'd seen many acupuncture cases of mine when he had been a school pupil, applying to get onto the veterinary course. Despite acupuncture not being in his university curriculum, he said he had been inspired to train in it after qualifying, so hopefully he will be able to answer his own questions, including whether acupuncture can help horses with keloid scarring, as it can in humans!

Lewis now knows there is science behind acupuncture, as does dentist Aleks; even so, Aleks told a friend of hers that she was coming to me for 'hippy treatment', which reveals how some people still perceive acupuncture. We laughed about it because she has seen the benefits to her dog Peanut and her husband Bryan (back in Chapter 12). Aleks' problem was a different challenge – could acupuncture, by influencing the immune system, reduce the severity of the laryngitis she develops every December when she loses her voice and has to take days off work? We found the answer to be yes!

October 2019—Three cases (feline, canine and human)

Cat Maisie calmly viewed her surroundings as she sat on her towel on the consulting room table, unaware of the needles in her back. I talked to her and stroked the long grey fur around her ears every now and again. She was purring. Owner Anna gazed at her lovingly and with pride. She smiled and commented, "I think Maisie likes coming for acupuncture. She has always wailed and hissed before at the vets." It feels as if all three of us are smiling.

At home, Maisie's back was better; she could once again reach her cat perch at the window and thus avoided the trauma of being dosed with a daily tramadol tablet.

Bichon Frise Charlie couldn't wait to come into the consulting room. His bandy front legs will always look the same because of his congenital elbow dysplasia and arthritis, but his owner Jill said he had been transformed ever since his first acupuncture session. Now he rarely limps on his front left leg, and is more agile and sprightly, and his walks have doubled in length. Charlie has always been agitated about coming to the vets, but Jill was stunned by his behaviour at his fourth acupuncture visit. She said, incredulously:

"I am at the vets, Charlie has tried to jump on your table, and now he's lying down on it!"

Back at home, Jill and her husband watched in amazement as Charlie raided his toy box, which he hadn't done in a very long time. Her husband even asked her if Charlie was getting some kind of injection – as well as the acupuncture – to explain the dramatic changes in him, but we know it is acupuncture alone! Being nine years old now, we are glad to have the option of acupuncture to help Charlie in the years ahead.

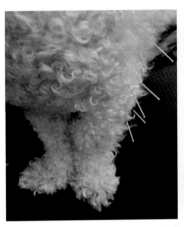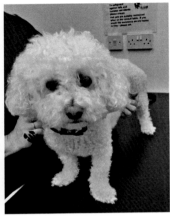

After acupuncture Charlie's elbows were no longer sore to touch.

Meanwhile Jennifer was travelling the forty-five mile stretch from Dundee to Dunfermline, to come to me for laser acupuncture. Two years previously her local hospital withdrew the option of this treatment, which had been making her life manageable. Since then, her doctors have struggled to find effective pain medication for her. She has suffered from chronic pain in her limbs for years due to a condition called CRPS (chronic regional pain syndrome), for which there is no standard treatment. It is early days yet, but at her last visit with me the swelling in her hands had markedly reduced and she was in less pain. She was in much better spirits and looking forward to starting a new job.

January 2020—An acupuncture boost

In contrast to Jennifer, Fiona had been coming to me for acupuncture and massage for thirteen years. We met when Fiona, then in her twenties, had been off work for six months due to post-viral fatigue and muscle pain. She was very low in spirits and frustrated by her lack of energy to be able to work, or to socialise and even to cope with simple daily tasks, so she was seeking ways to help herself. She responded to acupuncture very well, which allowed her to overcome the fatigue and pain, and so she was able to return to work. Since then, she has started a family. However, when she came back to me that January, she was struggling with chronic sinusitis and recurring infections, despite surgical intervention. While massage helped to soothe the build-up of shoulder tension, Fiona has always felt that acupuncture gives her a much-needed boost. And because of her word-of-mouth recommendations, both her brother and mother also came for treatment!

Fiona has recently reported having another 'boost'. After a discussion about recent publicity over how many Scots are low in vitamin D, and the effect this can have on the body including the immune system, a blood test revealed that she had low levels of the vitamin. Since taking an oral vitamin D spray she feels better and has far more energy. During the Covid-19 pandemic, early in 2021, the Scottish government published recommendations on vitamin D intake. They state:

> *... everyone aged five years and over should consider taking a daily supplement of vitamin D, particularly during the winter months (October to March).*

This has implications for many of us.

February 2020—A case of twitching buttocks

As I listened to a request to help someone out with their twitching buttocks, it crossed my mind that the call might be a hoax – but the person's voice was far too sincere for that. After over twenty years using acupuncture there are still surprises. Barbara was quite matter of fact about the muscles in her buttocks; they twitched for hours at a time – any time after teatime and into the night – and had been doing so since 1983!

I really couldn't believe what I was hearing. Her doctors had concluded that degeneration in her lower spine and the presence of cysts were irritating certain spinal nerves, but there wasn't a surgical option for her. She was in pain as well as suffering from the twitching. Four years of treatment with a Parkinson's disease medication, pramipexole, prescribed for restless legs, had not helped despite increasing the dose. When her consultant recommended that she stopped taking it, she had found it very difficult to do so. Thereafter she was only able to take paracetamol, and use a TENS machine (where patches are attached to the skin and an electrical current from a powerpack flows through the area of pain). This helped a little with the twitching, but for the spasms that came in the middle of the night she found what worked best was to apply pressure to them with a wooden spoon! They would eventually settle down enough for her to get some sleep, at least. Exercise and core strengthening had been recommended to her in the past, but she was a slim and fit yoga teacher!

While Barbara believed in acupuncture, she had been to several acupuncturists over the years and nothing had worked. I explained that I wouldn't be doing anything different unless we tried electro-acupuncture. In theory, if we could reproduce the twitching with an electric current it might switch off the unwanted flurry of messages from the nerves to her buttock muscles.

Barbara was more than happy to give it a go. From the start it was all very positive. During her first treatment I placed four needles, one at the centre of each buttock at point GB30 (Fig. 1), and the others nearer to the top of her pelvis. Barbara said it was certainly 'hitting the spot' and it felt good. She wished she had an electro-acupuncture machine at home! A month later, at the second treatment, I anxiously asked how she had been. No twitching for a whole week, she told me, and even when it felt as if it was going to start up again, it didn't! I was a bit disappointed that her pain was the same as before, but Barbara was absolutely delighted not to be pacing the floor at teatime or in the middle of the night. And she didn't need that wooden spoon anymore!

After five treatments Barbara said that the twitching was ninety-nine per cent better – that electro-acupuncture had transformed her life! She became calmer and appreciated the joy of being able to go out for a meal or to see a concert and sit still happily for hours. We plan to continue with electro-acupuncture and increase the interval between treatments if we can, but I do hope to do more to help with her pain.

As for myself, I feel humbled, yet again, as I endeavour to maintain an open mind and keep exploring what acupuncture can do. It is nearly twenty-one years since acupuncture entered my life. My acupuncture clinics for dogs, cats and humans continued – but what about the future of acupuncture?

— 18 —
The future of acupuncture

The medical arts of science and healing should be made available to people when they need them.

Aneurin Bevan (Minister of Health who launched the NHS in 1948)

I was amazed when I learned that scientists could measure changes taking place in the brains of meditating monks. A meditator may instinctively know that the effects are beneficial, but scientists like measurable effects. This has only been possible since methods were developed to detect changes in brain activity and measure the release of substances by the tissues of the brain.

At the time of writing this book, in 2019, the *NICE Guidelines* for the NHS in England and Wales advise on the use of therapies based on 'evidence-based recommendations developed by independent committees, including professionals and lay members, and consulted on by stakeholders'. They recommended acupuncture as an option for treating migraines and headaches. Acupuncture for treating back pain was first included in 2009, but was removed in 2016, which led to the withdrawal of acupuncture in some NHS clinics. While there is extensive research and positive results have been obtained for acupuncture – for both back pain and osteoarthritis of the knee – interpretation of the evidence varies and debate still rages among the healthcare decision-makers.

Acupuncture research is ongoing, however, despite difficulties in sourcing funds. At a BMAS conference in 2017, I and many others felt that things were gathering momentum. The conference topics included: acupuncture for pain control following caesarean section; the use of ear acupuncture for pain control; and its role in relieving exam anxiety. All fascinating subjects, but it was a particular man who captivated the audience – eighty-eight-year-old professor, Geoffrey Burnstock.

Professor Burnstock, who has since died, was world-renowned for his lifetime's research into pain, identifying neurotransmitters and receptors in the body that can be blocked by certain molecules to control pain. Although he was not involved with acupuncture, he theorised about the way it works. He believed it involves the release of a substance called adenosine triphosphate (ATP), part of the energy transport system within cells, which would explain why placing a needle in one part of the body can have distant effects on other areas, by acting on nerve receptors and pain-modulating nerves and interrupting pain pathways to the brain. His own work showed that such receptors vary according to our genes, and suggested that individual sensitivity to acupuncture depends on our genetic makeup. In future, GPs may be able to access our unique genetic data, and thus identify the diseases to which we may be more prone. Among other things, it will help reveal which treatments will suit each of us best, and that may include acupuncture.

At the 2018 BMAS conference, the topics on offer included the benefits of electro-acupuncture for osteoarthritis in the knee, and the release of endorphins – opiate-like substances we produce naturally (and the reason why opiate drugs have an effect on us). Jens Foell, a GP and lecturer with a special interest in patients with chronic pain, raised issues in his talk about how we are influenced by Eastern and Western belief systems. He suggested that there was far more to acupuncture treatment than the selection of points and needling techniques, including the context of the treatment and attitude and demeanour of the practitioner.

Then there was Vitaly Napadow, an associate professor at Harvard Medical School in the USA. He described the changes seen on functional MRI (fMRI) scans of the brain, that show in real-time how a patient reacts to a stimulus of any kind. For example, patients with carpal tunnel syndrome – a painful condition in which the median nerve at the wrist is trapped – showed a reduction in symptoms with acupuncture treatment. These changes were measurable using fMRI. We have a lot to look forward to as we gain a better understanding of the brain, its circuitry and wiring, which will enable us to see the precise effects of treatments like acupuncture.

Dr Carolyn Reubens, then the president of BMAS, described her success in establishing an acupuncture service for cancer patients. She enthused about its place alongside medication and psychological support for controlling cancer symptoms. I gathered from what she said that there was more hope in certain parts of the UK for developing acupuncture services through the private sector and social enterprises outwith the NHS. It seems that acupuncture services have been squeezed, with increasing pressure on the NHS because of an ageing population, and the support required for chronic illnesses, as well as a lack of funding. Furthermore, many people in positions of influence are still sceptical about its effectiveness.

It may be a simplistic view, but surely the NHS would benefit enormously, in terms of cost, if it could simply determine whether the consumption of medicines decreases in people who are treated with acupuncture. The use of acupuncture could result in some patients requiring fewer GP and hospital appointments and less prescribed medications. The issue is – as always – the problem of funding the research, especially as the drug industry would not be involved.

In both the veterinary and medical fields there is focus on evidence-based medicine in which treatments have been trialled and results published. However, much depends on the way a trial was run, and the number of variable factors involved, which means the results can be interpreted in different ways. And this applies to trials of pharmaceuticals, as much as any other intervention. The problem facing acupuncture is that it is often compared to a 'sham' procedure (like a placebo tablet in a drug trial), whereby some participants are treated with non-penetrating 'pretend' needles. However, even though the needles don't penetrate the skin, there is some mechanical stimulation of the area – the mere pressure of the needle on the surface of the skin can cause a local response and activate nerves and therefore have some kind of therapeutic effect. Many researchers don't believe this is suitable for comparison with the effect of penetrating needles. What is most relevant are the trials that compare real needles with drugs. Another complication is the wide variation in the teaching and methods of acupuncture in traditional Chinese and Western approaches. The UK Government review of the regulation and standardisation of the treatment was halted during the recession of 2008–09.

Sometimes a medicine can be successful without knowing exactly how it works, and there can be unforeseen side effects. While modern medicine has achieved so much, many people are looking for alternatives to drugs – primarily in the field of pain control – to avoid side effects. Let's not forget the issues arising from opiate dependency in some communities.

There has been much coverage in the press about opiate-abuse in the USA. The book *American Overdose: The Opioid Tragedy in Three Acts* by Chris McGreal (2018) gives a very readable but shocking explanation of the crisis, and includes evidence about how the over-prescription of inappropriately strong opiates has led to addiction in millions of Americans. In a review of the book in the *British Journal of General Practice* (see *Further reading*), Dr Jack Leach asked whether the US experience was relevant to the situation in the UK. He pointed out that in the UK there have been recent increases in the number of prescriptions and sales of over-the-counter opiate drugs, and an increase in the use of stronger ones, some of which are not backed up by evidence of their effectiveness in chronic pain. There has also been an increase in drug-related deaths. Dr Leach said that while pharmaceutical companies have less influence in the UK than in the US, their impact is still substantial; the irony is that some have gone on to promote new pharmaceuticals to counteract the addictive effects of the opiates!

With what we already know about addiction and side-effects from many painkillers, there is surely an even greater need to look for other options such as acupuncture. Craig's case, in Chapter 16, demonstrates how the use of acupuncture not only helps patients when all else has failed, but can be cost-saving to the NHS, in terms of GP time, the drugs, and the human cost of side effects. And it can mean that otherwise incapacitated people function properly again and may even return to work! If the benefits that Craig described are extrapolated to other people who respond to acupuncture, then the benefit to the nation would be inestimable.

Coincidentally, at the time of writing in 2019, trials were being conducted in Kentucky in an effort to combat the high incidence of opiate addiction, using a device designed in the 1970s by a Scottish surgeon, Dr Meg Patterson (who died in 2002). She trained in acupuncture while working in Hong Kong, where she was 'inspired' by opium addicts. Dr Patterson observed that their cravings for the drug either reduced or disappeared after electro-acupuncture. She went on to develop a battery-powered neuro-electric therapy (NET) machine, which uses tiny electrodes taped just behind the ears to send electrical pulses into the body. A documentary made in 2020, called *The Final Fix* (narrated by actor Ewan McGregor), tracked the experience of drug addicts who received NET and it concluded that the treatment is worthy of further consideration, despite having been dismissed for decades. The technique has been found to reduce cravings and withdrawal symptoms in a variety of addictions including smoking and alcohol and drug misuse. The theory is that it stimulates the brain to produce more endorphins. An article published in the *British Medical Journal* (2021) said that in 2018, drug users in Scotland had the highest death rate in Europe and there is need to develop public health policy to address this. Perhaps this may all contribute to the coming of a new age for acupuncture.

There are many similarities between the medical and veterinary worlds when it comes to increased use of the same old and stronger new medications, as well as the growing awareness of the importance of lifestyle. At a meeting in September 2019, sponsored by manufacturers of stance-analysers (weighing platforms), vet Professor Stuart Carmichael and the Radio Scotland vet Ross Allan – both experts in canine orthopaedics – reminded the vets who came to listen about the importance of lifestyle changes for animals with mobility problems. They advocated weight control and exercise, along with environmental modifications that are often overlooked. These things, and adjuncts like hydrotherapy, physiotherapy and acupuncture should be considered way before deciding to use strong pain medications. To me, their words reinforce what I have been trying to achieve through acupuncture, where my focus has, for so long, been on working with dogs and cats and humans …

Looking back over my long career, I can see why I am no longer a sceptic about acupuncture. I have learned so much from my animal and human patients and, despite my naysayer voice, become a complete convert after seeing with my own eyes its therapeutic effects. I feel fortunate to have had this opportunity when so many others haven't. Acupuncture became a routine procedure for me, and for my many patients, and in 2015 I decided to stop my routine veterinary work because I needed more time to meet the demand for acupuncture.

My use of acupuncture is only the tip of the iceberg in terms of its potential use in clinical practice. I never imagined I'd be able to use it in cases of anosmia or keloid scarring. I know some 'purists' in both Western and traditional Chinese acupuncture may question my methods – and my limitations – but I have always tried to apply the training I have received to deliver appropriate treatment to both my human and animal patients. However, the uses of acupuncture are so much wider! It can be used in cancer clinics and hospices for the control of symptoms such as nausea and vomiting as well as pain and for some side effects of chemotherapy such as hot flushes and peripheral neuropathy (pain and tingling in the hands and feet). It can be used for fertility problems and IVF, where it can stimulate uterine blood flow, for example; it can reduce morning sickness, and prepare the body for the birth process. I often get requests for help for the latter but always used to refer these women to a local, retired NHS midwife – a very experienced traditional Chinese acupuncturist. When she stopped practising, I began referring them to Susie Murphy at the Birkenshaw Clinic in Uddingston. Susie is an experienced BMAS acupuncturist and retired NHS midwife.

Acupuncture is increasingly used by vets who work at the 'coalface', as part of their routine treatment, and not necessarily in separate acupuncture clinics. It is also used in the pain clinics of some veterinary schools. But it still hasn't gained the recognition I believe it deserves, including that of the Royal College of Veterinary Surgeons. The availability of acupuncture is frankly a bit of a postcode lottery, and all depends on whether a vet – or a doctor – has encountered it themselves or the opportunity to train in its use has arisen. Health policy-makers really need to be on board with the technique, so that acupuncture becomes a universal option for all, that is integrated into mainstream human and veterinary medicine, and that is taught to some level in both vet and medical schools.

As you will know from reading this book, I have been hugely influenced by what I have witnessed throughout my career. While some people may discount the events in this book as 'anecdotal evidence', I believe there is real value in describing these events with various humans and animals with diverse problems. I acknowledge that acupuncture doesn't work for every person or every animal, but for so many it makes a great difference.

I hope that in the future medicine will become more integrative. There are signs that this is happening. I believe that acupuncture has an important role to play in our own and our pets' health, and will inevitably have the greater recognition it deserves.

I was once introduced to a retired GP, as a vet who treats animals and humans with acupuncture. This doctor remarked, "It makes sense. Humans are animals too".

I'm certainly not advocating that all vets should treat humans, but I do hope that the tales about the two-legged and four-legged patients that appear in this book demonstrate how much might be gained from treating both! I am always mindful that no treatment – including acupuncture – is a panacea but it is worthy of greater consideration for the health and welfare of all, especially in cases where there is no other option.

The tales in this book are, therefore, a celebration. A celebration of the help this gentle approach has given to my human, canine and feline patients.

And for those who haven't experienced acupuncture yet, I would urge you to seek it for yourself and your pet – then you can make up your own mind.

Epilogue

My husband Kenneth and I were visiting friends in New Zealand in 2020 when the Covid-19 pandemic hit, and we spent an extra four weeks there in level-four lockdown in Tauranga until our flight home to the UK. The virus, it seems, probably originated in a species of bat. This just underlines how inextricably linked we humans are with the animal kingdom. I am sure the concept of 'One Health' will only strengthen in the future, when we will place greater importance on understanding the cause and effect of our actions on the animal kingdom, the environment and human health as a consequence.

My friends, GP Liz, vet Angus and I have all had the same thought. We now wonder, following the success with acupuncture in restoring Dawn's post-viral loss of smell and taste (Chapter 15), whether acupuncture might help restore the loss of smell and taste in people for whom it persists after being infected by Covid-19. And what about the effect acupuncture could have on the immune system for post-viral fatigue and other symptoms included in what is known as 'long Covid'? After all my years with acupuncture, it feels like this ancient art of medicine should be explored yet further to deal with our very modern problems, especially where there may be limited or no conventional treatment options.

Several animals in these stories have now passed away, including my own cat Guinness (pictured here and on page 127). After a liver tumour had taken its toll, I had to put him to sleep late one Saturday night. Earlier on that day he had still managed to climb the stairs, to lie in his favourite spot. Although I never knew his age exactly, it was a grand age.

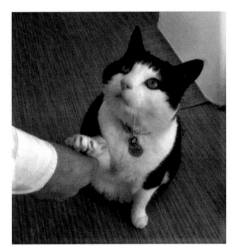

Guinness asking for a treat.
He loved his food!

I was also very sorry that I couldn't see Kola (Chapter 14) because of returning from abroad and the lockdown restrictions.

Just a few days before I finished writing the first draft of this book (in May 2020), she was put peacefully to sleep at the Dick vet school, a month short of fifteen years of age, following nearly ten years of acupuncture. We will never know what difference acupuncture made to her life, but her owners, Alison and Paul, never for one minute imagined they would have her for so long. She had received much medical help, it is true, but they don't think she'd have coped with it all without acupuncture.

All through lockdown, I was impatient to catch up with the many requests I received during that time. Regretfully some of the humans and animals, like Pickles, Barney, Marge and Sylvia, had to miss their regular sessions for acupuncture and laser treatment, and they had to go back on to medication. In contrast, I was comforted to know that Paolo was still happily running around on the beach!

It wasn't until July 2020 that restrictions relaxed enough for me to see my animal patients again – but not the humans. The pandemic changed all clinical practice significantly, and some of those changes may be permanent.

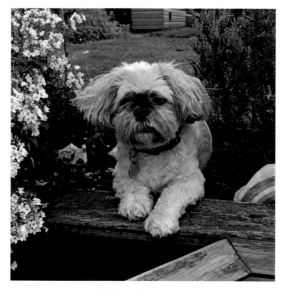

Pickles in lockdown.

NICE shines the light on acupuncture

I was delighted when a new set of NICE Guidelines were published in April 2021. They included the use of acupuncture for the treatment of 'chronic primary pain'. The guidelines stated:

"The committee made a recommendation to consider acupuncture or dry needling for chronic primary pain caveated by the factors likely to make the intervention cost effective."

This was great news, although some of the 'factors' are very limiting and any changes in regulations in the NHS tend to take some time to filter down, but they certainly give a green light for acupuncture to be made more available to patients with certain conditions and may lead to more funding for staff to train in acupuncture.

Also, the guidelines relate only to the NHS in England and Wales, but they will affect decisions made in Scotland, too. There is still a long way to go ...

After the guidelines were issued, BMAS published a book called *Western Medical Acupuncture Protocols for Chronic Pain*. It is a manual for people trained in acupuncture to refer to when considering the use of the therapy for treating certain painful conditions such as fibromyalgia and osteoarthritis, and areas including the head, neck, shoulder, arm, back and leg. It draws on a large body of published evidence.

I am sure Aneurin Bevan was not thinking of acupuncture when he said at the launch of the NHS in 1948: "The medical arts of science and healing should be made available to people when they need them".

I do believe that acupuncture has a role to play and should be available now and in the future. No doubt Mr Bevan could not have envisaged the expansion of the NHS to the extent it has, with the advances in technology and array of pharmaceuticals available, never mind the developments in veterinary medicine! We now have a range of options for pain control, for example, and the end of 2021 saw the arrival of a monthly injectable treatment of monoclonal antibodies for the pain of osteoarthritis in dogs and cats – ahead of a human formulation! While new treatment options will continue to appear, I believe there will always be a place for acupuncture.

During lockdown, GP Liz Phillips, ENT consultant David Walker, patient Dawn Busby and I wrote a letter to the journal *Acupuncture in Medicine*, relating to the successful treatment of Dawn's loss of smell and taste (Chapter 15). It was published in the summer of 2021. Her story is out there now – in the academic domain – where it may help other patients who have lost their smell and taste.

Liz told me that being involved with this book rekindled her belief in acupuncture in general practice! She joined an NHS long-Covid group and thinks that perhaps the experience and research of anosmia and acupuncture may influence some decision-making here. She also embarked on a review of chronic pain, especially in fibromyalgia, with the aim of reducing patients' medication burden using acupuncture and hypnotherapy.

I also reflected on what to do with any profits made from this book. For every sale, a donation will be made to the charity Mission Rabies (www.missionrabies.com). Their aim is to eradicate human deaths from bites from rabid animals by using vaccines to prevent the disease in domestic animals. It feels appropriate to support the concept of 'One Health' in this way, to reduce suffering caused by another virus. By reading this book, you are supporting this worthwhile cause, and between us we can make a difference.

As I approached my sixtieth birthday, amid the imposed Covid-19 restrictions that reduced my workload considerably, I wondered about retiring from practice. I would miss all my patients, of course, and was concerned about what arrangements could be made for them. My human patients could be referred for acupuncture with BMAS-trained nurse, Sharon Doherty, who I knew from courses we'd attended together. She had her own private clinic in another GP practice in Dunfermline and was more than happy to oblige. I knew some patients would miss their massages from me, but they would be in good hands with Sharon. My animal cases were more of a worry, however – the owners would have much further to travel to find a veterinary acupuncturist and I didn't want to let them down.

But by meaningful coincidence, after only a week of pondering, I met vet Amy Greenhill. She was working at the St Clair practice, was trained in acupuncture, and had run a clinic in England. She approached me for advice, about moving from full-time locum work to develop her interest in acupuncture. It all fell into place for both of us and shortly after, Amy took over my veterinary clinics.

And after referring cases to me for so long, and being such an enthusiast about what she sees as 'my thing', Rachel Rogers now provides her own acupuncture service at Inglis Vets. She is also a clinical tutor in practice for final-year Dick Vet students; the fact that the students will have the opportunity to see acupuncture *in situ* is another plus.

Arrangements in place, I made the transition into retirement in September 2020 – although it felt really good when I was called back to the clinic for a few weeks to cover their animal cases! I know I'm going to miss seeing all these 'furries' as often as I'd like to, but another book beckons, and I need the generous time that comes with retirement (in theory!) to write it.

Kenneth and I welcomed two new kittens, Hamish and Fergus, into our home at the start of 2021. They were rescued at five-weeks of age, when their mother abandoned them. Vet Rachel gave them their vaccinations and sent a photo my way; they were four months old when they came to us. And what a joy they are – and a reminder of how simple life can be if you are lucky enough to have a place to call home and have your health.

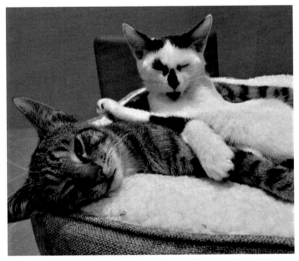

Hamish and Fergus who very quickly made themselves at home!

In July 2021, a statue of 'Street Cat Bob' was unveiled in London. The story of James and Bob is unique – a *must* read – and the statue is a poignant symbol of the importance of the very close relationships we can have with animals.

About the Author

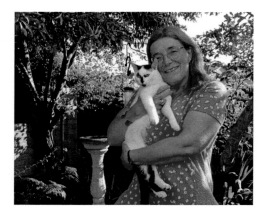

Dr Jane Hunter (pictured here with Fergus) is a veterinary surgeon who has had a varied career in different branches of the profession since qualifying from Glasgow University Veterinary School in 1983. She began in practice in the UK and Australia, completed a PhD and worked in the diagnosis of farm animal disease in the Scottish Borders, before becoming a lecturer in New Zealand.

In 1999 she returned home to Fife, Scotland and vet practice in Dunfermline. Having attended a lecture on acupuncture, despite initially being sceptical, she was inspired to train with the British Medical Acupuncture Society (BMAS) and was awarded their Diploma in 2006. Jane has been treating dogs, cats and humans with acupuncture for over twenty years and is passionate about integrating its use alongside conventional veterinary and human medicine.

Jane has always been fascinated by the human–animal bond, and interested in health and fitness. She lives in Dunfermline with her husband and two rescue cats, and has two grown-up step-children.

Glossary of terms

ABVA Association of British Veterinary Acupuncturists

AIM *Acupuncture in Medicine*, the international, peer-reviewed journal of BMAS on Western Medical Acupuncture

ataxia unsteady gait due to the brain's failure to regulate the body's posture and the strength and direction of limb movements

baltic very cold (Scots)

BMAS British Medical Acupuncture Society

cervical relating to the neck (see Figs 2 and 3)

chap knock (Scots)

Dick Vet University of Edinburgh Royal (Dick) School of Veterinary Studies

lumbar relating to the region of the back and side of the body between the lowest rib and the pelvis (see Figs 2 and 3)

MRI (magnetic resonance imagining) diagnostic scan for visualising soft tissue as well as bone

musculoskeletal relating to muscle and skeleton

neuropathic a disease or condition affecting the nervous system

NICE National Institute for Health and Care Excellence

NSAID (non-steroidal anti-inflammatory drugs) for use in animals and humans for post-operative pain and inflammation, and in acute and chronic musculoskeletal disorders; veterinary preparations include meloxicam, carprofen and robenacoxib

One Health: the concept that the health and wellbeing of people, animals and the environment are inextricably linked; professionals from these areas work together to effect best change and protection

opiate: a group of drugs derived from opium (includes synthetic 'opioid' drugs that have similar effects)

sacral: related to the sacrum, where fused vertebrae articulate with the lumbar vertebrae, coccyx and pelvis (see Figs 2 and 3)

side effect a secondary effects of a drug, usually an adverse one (but can occasionally be beneficial)

steroid a group of drugs with anti-inflammatory properties such as prednisolone

tammy Scots term for a woolly hat

thoracic relating to the chest (see Figs 2 and 3)

Useful links

Albavet
https://albavet.co.uk/our-practices/dunfermline

Association of British Veterinary Acupuncturists (ABVA)
www.abva.co.uk

British Acupuncture Council (BAC)
www.acupuncture.org.uk

British Medical Acupuncture Society (BMAS)
www.medical-acupuncture.co.uk

Canine arthritis management (CAM)
www.caninearthritis.co.uk

Dr Amy Greenhill at Forth View Veterinary Services
www.petacupuncture.co.uk

Dr Dan Keown
www.drdankeown.com

Dr Samantha Lindley at Glasgow Vet School
www.gla.ac.uk/schools/vet/sah/ourstaff/painclinic/samanthalindley

Inglis Vets (Dr Rachel Rogers)
www.inglisvet.co.uk

Long View Veterinary Services (Dr Samantha Lindley)
https://www.longviewveterinaryservices.com

Mission Rabies charity
www.missionrabies.com

One Health Centre (Africa)
www.ilri.org/research/facilities/one-health-centre

New Park Medical Practice (Sharon Doherty, BMAS acupuncturist)
https://www.newparkmedicalpractice.nhs.scot

St Clair Veterinary Group
https://www.stclairvet.co.uk

The Birkenshaw Clinic (Susie Murphy BMAS acupuncturist)
https://thebirkenshawclinic.com

Further reading

Anderson B (2010) *Stretching: 30th Anniversary Edition*. Shelter Publications.

Baldry PE (1998) *Acupuncture, Trigger Points and Musculoskeletal Pain* (2nd edn). Churchill Livingstone.

Bowen J (2012) *A Street Cat Named Bob*. Hodder.

British Journal of General Practice (2019) *Book review: American Overdose: The Opioid Tragedy in Three Acts* (by Chris McGreal). Available at: https://bjgp.org/content/69/682/251.

Christie B (2021) Record drug deaths need radical response, says Scottish college. *British Medical Journal* 2021;372:n593. Abstract available at https://dx.doi.org/10.1136/bmj.n593 BMJ 2021;372N593.

Connolly B (2010) *Journey to the Edge of the World*. Headline.

Cummings M, Lawler D, Sheikh A (2021) *Western Medical Acupuncture Protocols for Chronic Pain*. British Medical Acupuncture Society.

Doidge N (2008). *The Brain That Changes Itself: Stories of Personal Triumph from the Frontiers of Brain Science*. Penguin Books.

Doidge N (2016). *The Brain's Way of Healing*. Penguin Books.

Filshie H, White A (eds) (2001) *Medical Acupuncture: A Western Scientific Approach*. Churchill Livingstone.

Gunn CC (2002) *The Gunn Approach to the Treatment of Chronic Pain*. Churchill Livingstone.

Hecker HU, Steveling A, Peuker E, *et al.* (2000) *Pocket Atlas of Acupuncture and Trigger Points*. Thieme.

Hunter J (2011) Acupuncture for keloid scar. *Acupuncture in Medicine* 29(1):2.

Hunter JEB, Phillips ME, Walker FDL, Busby D (2021) Post-viral olfactory dysfunction treated with acupuncture. *Acupuncture in Medicine* 39(6). Available at: https://doi.org/10.1177/09645284211026315.

Keown D (2014) *The Spark in the Machine.* Singing Dragon.

Keown D (2018) *The Uncharted Body: A New Textbook of Medicine.* Original Medicine Publications.

Lindley S, Cummings M (2006) *Essentials of Western Veterinary Acupuncture.* Blackwell Publishing.

McGreal C (2018) *American Overdose: The Opioid Tragedy in Three Acts.* Guardian Faber.

NICE (2021) *Chronic pain (primary and secondary) in over 16s: assessment of all chronic pain and management of chronic primary pain. Guideline NG193.* Available at: https://www.nice.org.uk/guidance/ng193/chapter/rationale-and-impact#acupuncture-for-chronic-primary-pain-2

Schoen AM (1995) *Love, Miracles and Animal Healing.* Simon and Schuster.

Scottish Government (2021) *Vitamin D: advice for all age groups.* Available at: https://www.gov.scot/publications/vitamin-d-advice-for-all-age-groups

Travell JG, Simons DG (1998) *Travell and Simons' Myofascial Pain and Dysfunction: The Trigger Point Manual.* Lippincott, Williams &Wilkins.

World Health Organization (2019) *Traditional, complementary and integrative medicine.* Available at: https://www.who.int/health-topics/traditional-complementary-and-integrative-medicine#tab=tab_1

World Health Organization (2019) *Rabies.* Available at: https://www.who.int/news-room/fact-sheets/detail/rabies

Yellowlees W (1993) *Doctor in the Wilderness.* Pioneer.